DEEP TISSUE MASSAGE TREATMENT

A Handbook of Neuromuscular Therapy

Enrique Fabian Fernandez, NMT
Corporate Director of Education
Premier Education Group
Springfield, Massachusetts

MOSBY
ELSEVIER

MOSBY
ELSEVIER

11830 Westline Industrial Drive
St. Louis, Missouri 63146

DEEP TISSUE MASSAGE TREATMENT: A HANDBOOK OF NEUROMUSCULAR THERAPY

ISBN-13: 978-0-323-03734-1
ISBN-10: 0-323-03734-8

Notice

Knowledge and best practice in this field are constantly changing. As new research and experience broaden our knowledge, changes in practice, treatment and drug therapy may become necessary or appropriate. Readers are advised to check the most current information provided (i) on procedures featured or (ii) by the manufacturer of each product to be administered, to verify the recommended dose or formula, the method and duration of administration, and contraindications. It is the responsibility of the practitioner, relying on their own experience and knowledge of the patient, to make diagnoses, to determine dosages and the best treatment for each individual patient, and to take all appropriate safety precautions. To the fullest extent of the law, neither the Publisher nor the Author assumes any liability for any injury and/or damage to persons or property arising out of or related to any use of the material contained in this book.

The Publisher

ISBN-13: 978-0-323-03734-1
ISBN-10: 0-323-03734-8

Publishing Director: Linda Duncan
Acquisitions Editor: Kellie White
Developmental Editor: Jennifer Watrous
Editorial Assistant: Elizabeth Clark
Publishing Services Manager: Melissa Lastarria
Design Direction: Amy Buxton

Printed in Canada

Last digit is the print number: 9 8 7 6 5 4 3 2 1

This book is dedicated to the thousands of hands willing and not afraid to make a positive change in this world; to my wife and friend, Francis; and my children, Andrew, Joshua, and Matthew, for being my daily inspiration to be a better person; and to Jennifer Watrous and Kellie White for their efforts and support on making this dream a reality.

Foreword

In my 20 years as a massage therapy educator, I have seen an explosion in the acceptance and popularity of massage therapy. What was once viewed as a self-indulgent luxury for the wealthy is now understood to be therapeutically beneficial for everyone. Once restricted to spas, cruise ships, and resorts, massage therapy is now commonly found in physicians' offices, physical therapy centers, and hospitals. Even in our private practices, clients do not come in only to be de-stressed. Increasingly, they enter our office asking if massage therapy can help them with their headaches or low back pain; or lessen the pain and stiffness of whiplash caused by a car accident.

In short, clients are increasingly seeking out massage as a treatment for specific pathologic conditions from which they suffer. For this reason, massage therapy is now clearly recognized as a member of complementary and alternative medicine (CAM). While I firmly believe that all massage is therapeutic, when massage therapy is applied for the treatment of a specific condition, it is often called *therapeutic massage*. Other terms used synonymously are *clinical massage* and *medical massage*; and when the condition being treated is musculoskeletal in nature, the term *orthopedic massage* is often used. Regardless of the name that we assign it, massage therapy that is oriented at treating specific pathologic conditions of the body is becoming more and more popular and requires a specific knowledge and skill set on the part of the massage therapist.

This is where Fabian Fernandez's book, *Deep Tissue Massage Treatment*, is so valuable and needed. This book is divided into three parts. Part One of the book begins by addressing concepts of assessment and continues by describing how to apply common deep tissue techniques such as trigger point sustained compression, friction, and myofascial release. Part Three covers stretches that can be used in conjunction with the deep tissue techniques presented in the book. Part Two comprises the bulk of the book and covers 24 of the most common conditions that a therapist will see in practice. Thoracic outlet syndrome, lateral epicondylitis (tennis elbow), low back pain, piriformis syndrome, and plantar fasciitis are just a few examples of the conditions covered. In each case, the condition is explained, and indications and contraindications for treatment are given. However, the strength of this book is rooted in the deep tissue treatment protocols that are presented. For each pathologic condition, a step-by-step treatment protocol is explained and demonstrated in clear and easy-to-follow photographs. Anticipating the dynamic nature of massage therapy treatment, this book comes with an added bonus: a companion DVD that contains over 1 hour of video demonstrating the treatment protocols of the book.

Something I particularly admire about the book and DVD is the fine demonstration of body mechanics that Fabian Fernandez uses when demonstrating these treatment protocols. All too often, therapists try to "muscle" deep tissue work instead of learning to apply it using efficient body mechanics. The key to working smart instead of working hard is to employ the type of body mechanics that Fabian Fernandez consistently demonstrates. This will lead to both longevity in practice and more satisfied clients!

Regarding application, this book was designed for dual use. It is ideal as a core curriculum textbook, fitting nicely into the curriculum of a therapeutic/medical/clinical/orthopedic massage course, and its spiral bound design allows for easy use in the classroom. Further, each chapter contains an outline of the chapter information along with a list of key terms and learning objectives. There is also a comprehensive glossary of terms. Beyond classroom use, this book is a valuable reference book for practicing massage therapists who would like to begin applying deep tissue techniques on their clients.

While I recognize and appreciate the application of massage therapy in all arenas, I firmly believe that clinically applied therapeutic massage will only continue to grow in the future. Therefore, for anyone looking to practice deep tissue therapeutic massage, I strongly recommend this book. It will make an invaluable addition to your library!

Joseph E. Muscolino, DC
Instructor, Connecticut Center for Massage Therapy
Westport, Connecticut
Owner, The Art and Science of Kinesiology
Redding, Connecticut

PREFACE

In the many roads that life has taken me on I have discovered this: in order to make the transition from student to professional, students need a well thought-out, structured, basic starting point. They will find that in this book–a starting point to transition good therapists into *great* therapists.

I have been truly privileged in my life to have worked for many excellent companies such as Premier Education Group, Florida Career College, Career Education Corporation (CEC), Corinthian Colleges Inc. (CCI), Ultrasound Diagnostic Schools, and National School of Technology, as well as being an evaluator for accrediting agencies such as The Accrediting Council for Independent Colleges and Schools (ACICS) and Accrediting Bureau of Health Education Schools (ABHES). This experience has helped me understand the impact that a well thought-out educational process has on a student. Therefore, this book is tailored for students and therapists willing to take their massage practice to a whole new level and truly make a difference.

Deep Tissue Massage Treatment provides treatments for the 24 most common pathologies a massage therapist might encounter in the field. These treatment routines are designed to provide a treatment road map by which students and therapists learn step-by-step treatments to effectively help their clients in the pursuit of personal physical improvement.

Presented in a clear and easy-to-use format, this book provides basic assessment of neuromuscular conditions and an overview of techniques specific to deep tissue massage. The most commonly used techniques are covered with illustrations and instructions for performing techniques. The bulk of the book presents treatment routines for the 24 most commonly encountered neuromuscular conditions. Routines are outlined step-by-step and clearly describe exactly what therapists need to do to treat a particular condition. Furthermore, this handbook includes an alert icon that highlights specific precautions a therapist must take on particular areas.

This handbook is the first text on the market that delineates step-by-step deep tissue treatment routines. Neuromuscular conditions discussed include, but are not limited to: carpal tunnel syndrome, tennis and golfer's elbow, frozen shoulder, rotator cuff dysfunctions, thoracic outlet syndrome, whiplash, migraines, kyphosis, lordosis, scoliosis, fibromyalgia, sciatica, and temporal mandibular joint disorder (TMJD). Each chapter on conditions follows a template with a definition of the condition, a list of associated symptoms, indications and/or contraindications for massage, and a specific treatment. Treatments are heavily illustrated with numerous photos of each technique and routine. Photos of indicated stretches accompany this handbook to assist a therapist on proper application. The spiral bound edition makes it easier for the therapist to utilize the handbook while performing the techniques. The companion DVD demonstrates techniques and routines from each chapter.

Deep Tissue Massage Treatment: A Handbook of Neuromuscular Therapy is a must-have for therapists, students, and instructors. Students will enjoy learning through visual (text and pictures) and auditory (DVD) processes. Instructors will enjoy standardization across the curriculum when teaching these treatment routines. Practitioners will have the benefit of successfully implementing proven treatment routines.

Readers: Please note that this book is technique-oriented; therefore the draping in some of the pictures appears the way it does in an effort to make the techniques more visible and to clearly demonstrate *how* a technique should be performed. Proper draping procedures should be observed at all times when performing these techniques. At no time should draping be compromised.

Fabian Fernandez

Contents

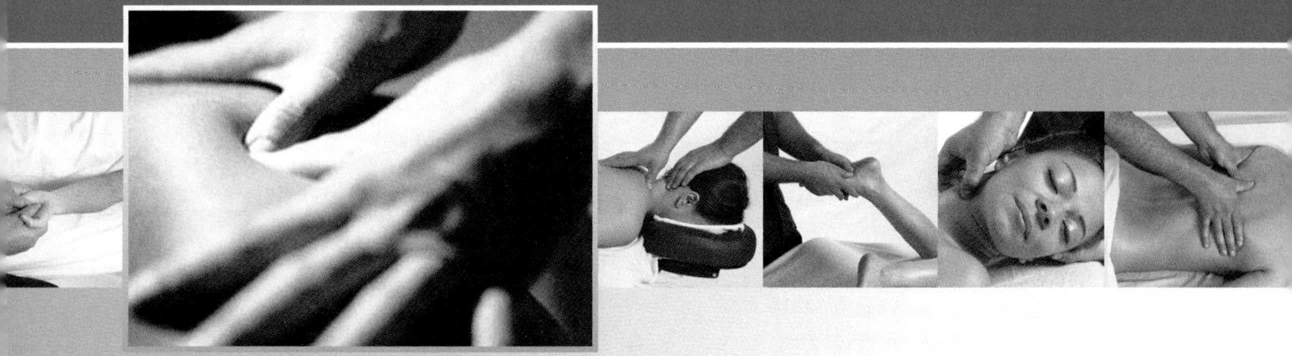

PART ONE

BASIC ASSESSMENT AND TECHNIQUES

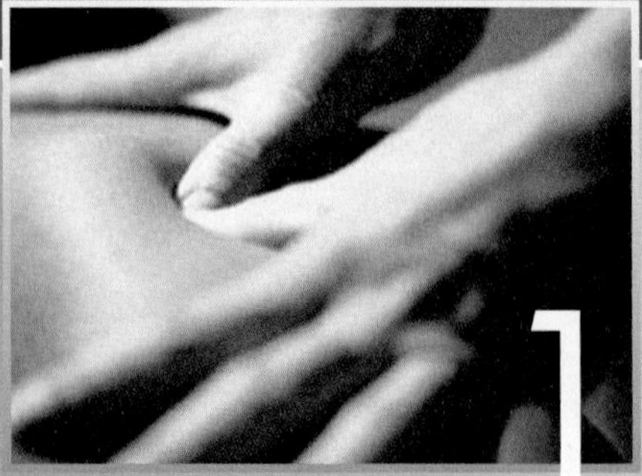

CHAPTER 1

ASSESSMENT

OUTLINE

Gait patterns
Assessment
Consultation
Definitions

KEY TERMS

Gait cycle
Stance phase
Heel strike
Mid-stance
Push-off
Swing phase
Painful-knee gait
Coxalgic gait
Sacroiliac gait
Hemiplegic's gait
Flexed-hip gait
Parkinson's gait
Client history
Ectomorphic
Mesomorphic
Endomorphic
Interview
Evaluation
Diagnosis
Prognosis
Intervention
Outcomes

OBJECTIVES

Upon completion of this chapter the reader will have the information necessary to:

1 **Define "normal gait"**
2 **Identify variations between the stance and swing phase**
3 **Describe differences between Parkinson's gait, flexed-hip gait, hemiplegic's gait, sacroiliac gait, coxalgic gait, and painful-knee gait**
4 **Understand various requirements needed for the observation, interview, and palpation stage**
5 **List specific requirements of the various interview stages**

GAIT PATTERNS

The following are some of the most common gait patterns a therapist will encounter in his or her day-to-day work with clients.

NORMAL GAIT

The **gait cycle** is the time interval between successive heel strikes of the same foot. The normal gait cycle consists of two major phases:

The **stance phase** is composed of three fluid movements. It begins with the **heel strike**, when the heel of the foot strikes the ground. It is followed by **mid-stance,** when the sole of the foot is flat on the ground and the body weight is directly over the leg. The last movement is **push-off**, when the heel of the leg lifts from the ground and the ball of the foot pushes the body forward. At this moment, the body is propelled forward by the action of the calf muscles and hyperextension of the hip.

The **swing phase** begins when the toes leave the ground and the leg has been brought forward; it ends when the heel strikes the ground again. During this phase, the leg should move rapidly to ready itself for the next heel strike. This is achieved by flexing the knee and hip, in order to clear the ground, as it is brought forward past the other leg. The swing phase ends at the exact moment of the heel strike, beginning stance phase again.

In combination with the leg movement, the pelvis rotates (in general, 6-8 degrees) around the spine in the transverse plane. The rotation comes to a complete stop at the exact time of the heel strike. As a person's full weight is placed on the leg in the mid-stance phase, rotation of the pelvis in the horizontal plane is reversed. As the opposite leg goes into the swing phase, the pelvis on the same side starts to rotate forward. The shoulder girdle imitates the hip by applying the same movement, but in reverse order. On the side where the pelvis rotates forward, the shoulder rotates backward.

There is one period in the gait cycle in which there is double support (two extremities are in contact with the ground at the same time). This occurs between the toe push-off on one side and the heel strike and mid-stance phase on the other. The length of time of double support is directly related to the speed a person is walking. As walking speed decreases, the length of time in double support increases. As walking speed increases, double support decreases. As walking speed increases to running speed, double support disappears entirely.

A person's gait will inevitably be altered with age. This occurs due to decreased ligament and muscle elasticity, including loss of joint surface smoothness. Changes in the neurological system also contribute to gait alterations. As a person gets older, his or her gait loses its "effortless" appearance. Certain diseases of the nervous and musculoskeletal systems may also cause gait deviations. One such ailment, frequently found among the elderly, is osteoarthritis of the hip joint, which generally results in a **painful-knee** or **coxalgic gait**.

PAINFUL-KNEE GAIT

A stiff or painful knee can be caused by osteoarthritis or other joint disorders. To protect the knee, a person will unconsciously contract the quadriceps to suppress any motion in the knee. The client therefore assumes an outward rotation of the affected extremity, resulting in a duck-like walk. The medial aspect of the leg and foot are pointed in the direction of forward motion. Therefore flexion and extension in the knee are avoided, and the entire sole of the foot can be placed on the ground, potentially resulting in an increased rotation of the pelvis.

COXALGIC GAIT

In osteoarthritis of the hip, the smooth head of the femur becomes uneven, restricting the motion of the hip joint (the motion of the femoral head in the acetabulum), making the joint restricted and painful. This is especially evident in the swing phase, when the hip and knee have to be flexed to bring the leg forward and in front of the other foot. The hyperextension of the hip at the end of the stance phase may be diminished; hence, the step becomes shorter. To enable the swing-phase leg to clear the ground in a very severe restriction of hip flexion, a person will lift the stance-phase leg up on the toes. The width of the step is reduced, depending on the degree of abduction limitation. Components of the normal gait that may be increased in the painful-knee or coxalgic gait are flexion and extension of the lumbar spine and backward and forward tilting of the pelvis. The lateral shift of the trunk is oftentimes increased, mainly with one-sided hip pain and restriction.

SACROILIAC GAIT

Motion between the sacrum and the iliac bone can be observed during normal gait. Both bones are firmly connected to each other. However, some motion during walking occurs in this area. Individuals who have any affliction or disorder in the sacroiliac joint tend to walk slightly bent forward with decreased motion of the pelvis. This results in restricted pelvic movement, followed by shorter steps.

HEMIPLEGIC'S GAIT

Often seen in elderly clients, this gait is usually caused by neurological accidents, such as stroke. Spasticity often appears in four to six weeks after the stroke, resulting in a partial or complete loss of movement and often resulting in severe gait deviations. When the hemiplegia is on the right side, arm swing on the right is lost. The client's arm dangles if it is flaccid, or it stays in a flexed-elbow position if spasticity has set in. To clear the ground during the swing phase, the hip has to be abducted as trunk flexion of the healthy side assists in gaining some elevation and momentum of the pelvis on the affected side. In this case there is minimal stride and the client walks on the outside of the affected foot, preventing the heel from touching the ground. In an effort to thrust the other leg forward, a person often pushes up on the healthy side by elevating the heel, resulting in further damage and degeneration to the foot, leg, hip, and spine.

FLEXED-HIP GAIT

In general, individuals who have flexion contractures of the hip-joint capsule have flexed-hip joint. Hip flexion contracture is frequently found in individuals who must sit for long periods of time due to pain in the lower extremities. Hip-joint dysfunction can also be caused by nerve compression, impingement, or neuromuscular dysfunction, among other causes.

PARKINSON'S GAIT

Parkinson's disease has a major effect on the central nervous system and on a person's gait. Most often found in elderly individuals, this ailment is often treated with drug therapy. A person who has Parkinson's disease stands with a slightly forward-flexed trunk and flexed knees and hips; there is often a continuous tremor throughout the body. In ambulation (walking), there is usually

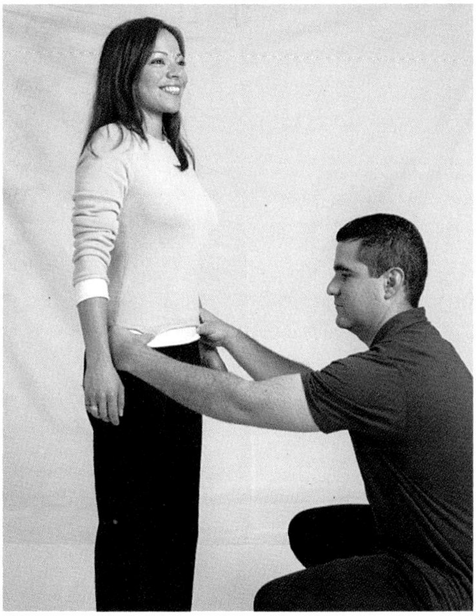

FIGURE 1-1 ■ Check for asymmetry between right and left anterior superior iliac spine.

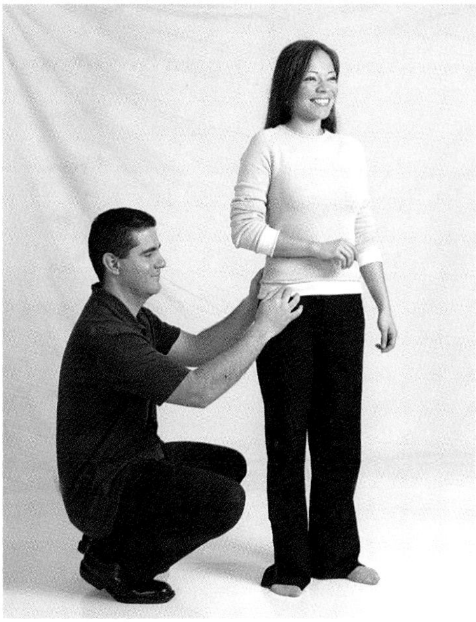

FIGURE 1-2 ■ Check for angle between anterior superior iliac spine and posterior superior iliac spine.

no arm swing and the trunk swings from right to left in a block motion. Gait deviation depends upon severity, intensity, and persistence of the disease.

ASSESSMENT

OBSERVATION

The therapist must observe the following:
(Figures 1-1, 1-2, 1-3, 1-4, and 1-5)

Overall Posture

1. Head and neck posture
2. Height of shoulders
3. Facial expression during different movements
4. Asymmetry of stance
5. Contours and landmarks (such as "love handles")
6. Areas of spasm

Body Type

1. **Ectomorphic:** thin body
2. **Mesomorphic:** muscular body
3. **Endomorphic:** heavy body

Gait and Ambulatory Patterns

Attitude

Is the client tense, stressed, or bothered?

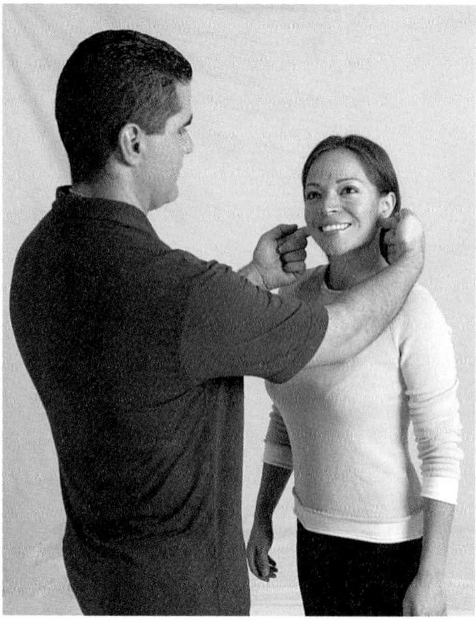

FIGURE 1-3 ■ Compare height of right and left mastoid process.

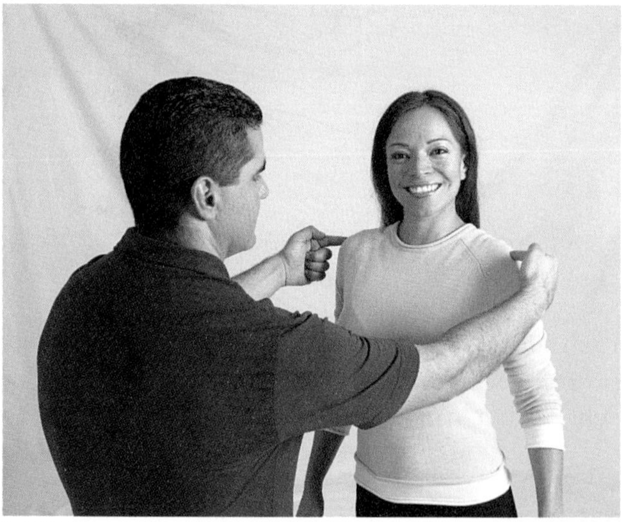

FIGURE 1-4 ■ Compare right and left shoulder height.

Spinal Posture

Does the client display signs of kyphosis, scoliosis, or lordosis?

Body Compensation

Does the body reflect signs of compensation resulting from pain or injury?

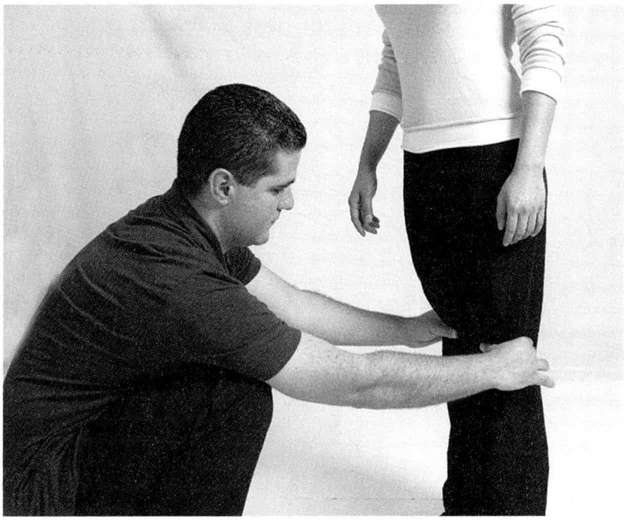

FIGURE 1-5 ■ Compare right and left knee height.

INTERVIEW (GATHERING INFORMATION)

The **interview** session must be as thorough as possible because even the smallest complaint, such as a heel spur, can cause a shift in gait or posture.

PALPATION

A therapist's livelihood depends on palpatory skills, including the correct application of palpation and proper interpretation of what is found.

CONSULTATION

PRELIMINARY INTERVIEW

Client History

A thorough **client history** must be taken to determine the type of massage treatment best suited for the individual. Questions about the type of work they do, accidents they have suffered, first pain occurrence, and physical sensations are all pieces of a larger puzzle waiting to be completed. Standard intake and SOAP (subjective, objective, assessment or analysis, and plan) note forms are provided for your convenience here (Figures 1-6 and 1-7).

Client's Medical History

To determine if massage is indicated or contraindicated, a thorough medical history of your client must be taken. This form is also available here (Figure 1-8).

Medical Intake and Release Form

Name_______________ Telephone_______________ Date of Birth_______________
Address_______________ City_______________ State___ Zip_______
Emergency Contact_______________ Telephone_______________
Occupation_______________ Height_______ Weight_______ ☐ Male ☐ Female

Are you in good health? ☐ Yes ☐ No
If "No" please explain_______________
Has there been any change to your health in the past year? ☐ Yes ☐ No
If "Yes" please explain_______________

Physician _______________ Telephone _______________

Mark Appropriate Stress Zones

Please circle the area of discomfort

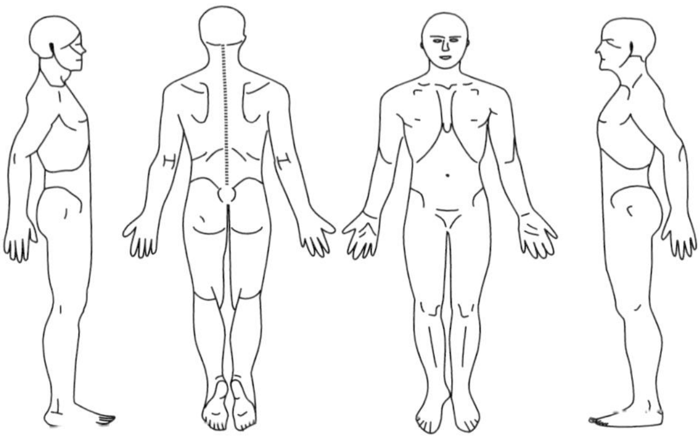

If answering "Yes" to any of the following questions, please explain in the space provided.

Are you currently taking any medication?	☐Yes ☐No	Do you bruise easily?	☐Yes ☐No
Do you suffer from acne?	☐Yes ☐No	Do you suffer from heart disease?	☐Yes ☐No
Do you suffer from allergies?	☐Yes ☐No	Do you have diabetes?	☐Yes ☐No
Do you suffer from arthritis?	☐Yes ☐No	Do you suffer from asthma?	☐Yes ☐No
Do you suffer from high blood pressure?	☐Yes ☐No	Do you have any blood disorder?	☐Yes ☐No
Do you suffer from epilepsy or seizures?	☐Yes ☐No	Do you have seborrhea?	☐Yes ☐No
Do you suffer from claustrophobia?	☐Yes ☐No	Are you pregnant or nursing?	☐Yes ☐No
Do you have any contagious disease?	☐Yes ☐No	Do you wear contact lenses?	☐Yes ☐No
Do you have varicose or spider veins?	☐Yes ☐No	Have you ever had surgery?	☐Yes ☐No
Do you wear a pacemaker?	☐Yes ☐No	Do you have any herniated disks?	☐Yes ☐No
Do you suffer from chronic back pain?	☐Yes ☐No	Do you suffer from stress?	☐Yes ☐No

Are you wearing any patches?
Have you ever had or are you currently being treated for cancer? ☐Yes ☐No
Are you currently being treated by a physician for any condition? ☐Yes ☐No
Do you have any medical condition I should know about? ☐Yes ☐No
Are you taking any medications (including non-prescription)? ☐Yes ☐No
When was your last massage? _______________

Explain: _______________

Informed consent: The above information is accurate to the best of my knowledge and I freely give my permission to be massaged. I agree to inform the student and instructor of any experience of pain during the session. I understand that this is not a medical treatment and that this is not a substitute for medical diagnosis, treatment, or examination. Furthermore this is a session strictly designed to help students increase their Massage practice and experience. I understand that no inappropriate comments or conduct will be tolerated and that any indication of such will automatically end the session. I understand that all curtains will be drawn back (open) for instructional purposes while massage is in session and I further agree to hold harmless (Name of your School) and its subsidiaries, all management, students, volunteers, or campus where the massage is being conducted against any and all claims. I further understand that massage will be administered at the discretion of the instructor, program director, clinic director and/or lead instructor and any medical condition contraindicated to massage will disqualify me from participating in the massage practice.

_______________ _______________
Massage Recipient Date

_______________ _______________
Student Practicing Date

____
Instructor

FIGURE 1-6 ■ Sample intake form.

SESSION NOTES
SOAP CHARTING FORM

Client Name: ______________________ Date: __________

Practitioner Name: ______________________

Subjective

CLIENT STATUS

- **Information from client, referral source or reference books:**

1) Current conditions/changes from last session: ______________________

Objective

2) Information from assessment (physical, gait, palpation, muscle testing):

CONTENT OF SESSION

- **Generate goal (possibilities) from analysis of information in client status.**

1) Goals worked on this session. (Base information on client status this session and goals previously established in Treatment Plan):

What was done this session:

Analysis

RESULTS

- **Analyze results of session in relationship to what was done and how this relates to the session goals. (This is based on cause and effect of methods used and the effects on the persons involved).**

1) What worked/what didn't: (Based on measureable and objective Post Assessment)

Plan

PLAN: Plans for next session, what client will work on, what next massage will reassess and continue to assess: ______________________

CLIENT COMMENTS:

Time In: __________ Time Out: __________

Therapist signature: ______________________

FIGURE 1-7 ■ SOAP charting form. (From Fritz S: *Mosby's fundamentals of therapeutic massage*, ed. 3. St. Louis, 2004, Mosby.)

Client Health Record

Name: ______________________ Telephone: (____) __________ Date of Birth: ______________

Address: ______________________ City: __________ State: ______ Zip: __________

Referred by: ______________________ Telephone: (___) ______________

In case of emergency: ______________________ Telephone: (___) ______________

General & Medical Information

Occupation: ______________ Height: ________ Weight: __________ ❑ Male ❑ Female

Are you basically in good health? ❑ Yes ❑ No

Has there been any change to your health in the past year? ❑ Yes ❑ No

If so, please explain: ______________________

Physician: ______________________ Telephone: (___) ______________

If you answer "yes" to any of the following questions, please explain as clearly as possible.

Do you suffer from acne? ❑ Yes ❑ No

Do you have allergies? ❑ Yes ❑ No
Specify:
____

Do you have arthritis? ❑ Yes ❑ No

Do you have high blood pressure? ❑ Yes ❑ No
If yes, what medication are you taking?
____

Do you suffer from epilepsy or seizures? ❑ Yes ❑ No

Do you suffer from claustrophobia? ❑ Yes ❑ No

Do you have varicose veins or distended capillaries? ❑ Yes ❑ No

Do you have any contagious diseases? ❑ Yes ❑ No

Do you have heart disease? ❑ Yes ❑ No

Do you have diabetes? ❑ Yes ❑ No

Do you have asthma? ❑ Yes ❑ No

Have you ever had or are you being treated now for cancer? ❑ Yes ❑ No
Please explain:
____

Do you suffer from any blood disorder? ❑ Yes ❑ No

Do you have seborrhea? ❑ Yes ❑ No

Have you ever had surgery? ❑ Yes ❑ No
Please explain:
____

Are you pregnant or nursing? ❑ Yes ❑ No

Do you wear contact lenses? ❑ Yes ❑ No

Do you wear dentures? ❑ Yes ❑ No

Do you have a pacemaker? ❑ Yes ❑ No

Are you currently being treated by a physician for any condition? ❑ Yes ❑ No
Please explain:
____

Do you have any other medical condition I should know about?
____

Are you taking any medications (*including non-prescription drugs*)

❑ Birth Control Pills ❑ Diuretics
❑ Accutane ❑ Vitamins/Supplements
❑ Hormone Therapy ❑ Antibiotics
❑ Aspirin/Ibuprofen/Acetaminophen
❑ Vitamin A (topical or internal)

Are you using any of the following products?

❑ Renova ❑ Benzoyl Peroxide
❑ Glycolic Acid ❑ Retin-A

How much water do you drink a day? __________ glasses

Do you exercise regularly? ❑ Yes ❑ No

How would you describe your overall level of stress?
❑ Low ❑ Medium ❑ High

Comments: ______________________
____
____
____
____

Please take a moment to carefully read the information you have provided and sign where indicated. If you have a specific medical condition or specific symptoms, certain esthetic treatments may be contraindicated. A referral from your primary care provider may be required prior to service being rendered.

Client Signature: ______________________ Date: ______________

FIGURE 1-8 ■ Sample medical history form. (Copyright 2001 Associated Bodywork & Massage Professionals. All rights reserved. A sample form. Permission is hereby granted to reproduce this form in its entirety, including the copyright notice, for commercial or instructional use but not for resale.)

DEFINITIONS

All therapists must be familiar with the following terms:

- **Evaluation**–a process in which a licensed healthcare practitioner (physician, chiropractor, or physical therapist) makes a clinical judgment based on information gathered during the interview and examination

- **Diagnosis**–the decision reached at the end of the examination and evaluation, organized into defined clusters, syndromes or categories to help determine the most appropriate intervention strategies

- **Prognosis**–determination of the level of optimal improvement that might be attained through intervention and the amount of time required to reach that level.

- **Intervention**–purposeful and skilled interaction of the therapist with the client and, when appropriate, other individuals also involved in the client's care using various methods and techniques to produce changes in the condition that are consistent with the diagnosis and prognosis.

- **Outcomes**–result of client pain management, which includes remediation of functional limitation and disability, and optimization of client satisfaction, including primary or secondary prevention.

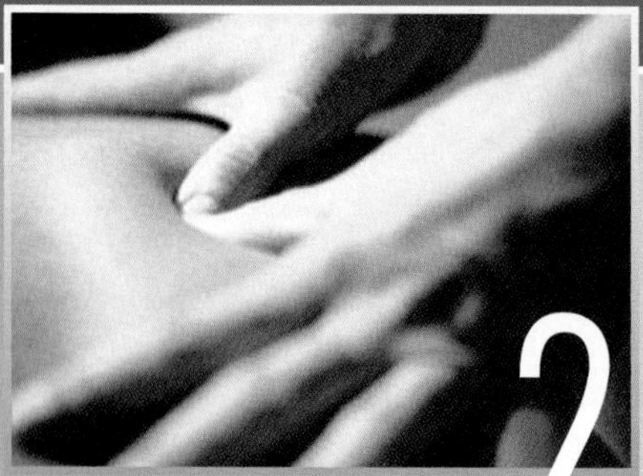

CHAPTER 2

TRIGGER POINT THERAPY

OUTLINE

Classification
Location
Palpation
Release Methods
Caution

KEY TERMS

Trigger point
Inactive trigger point
Active trigger point
Latent trigger point
Ischemic compression
Stretching

OBJECTIVES

Upon completion of this chapter the reader will have the information necessary to:

1 **Define trigger point therapy**
2 **Identify various trigger point classifications**
3 **Describe various palpation identifiers**
4 **Understand various trigger point release methods**
5 **List various trigger point techniques**

T**rigger point** is an area of high-nerve facilitation that is hyperirritable and painful when compressed, which may result in muscle dysfunction and/or chronic condition.

Most acute and all chronic neuromuscular conditions produce trigger points in the body. These trigger points represent a major cause of dysfunction and constant pain, which some clients refer to as "annoying pain." There has been an abundance of information, including various schools of thought, concerning trigger point techniques, pressure, and intensity. However, to simplify our understanding we will be analyzing the most basic techniques and classifications that will be needed for the treatments described in this book.

CLASSIFICATION

An **inactive trigger point** does not show local tenderness or refer pain when compressed; excess trigger point stimulation might activate this trigger point.

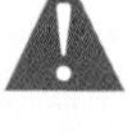

Icon represents an area where extreme caution should be used to avoid damage or compression to underlying or neighboring vessels.

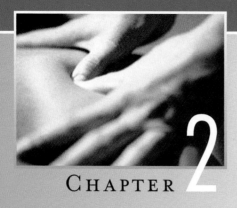

An **active trigger point**, when stimulated, refers pain and tenderness to another area of the body that is usually not associated by nerve or a dermatome segment.

A **latent trigger point** only exhibits pain when compressed and does not refer pain; it may or may not radiate pain around the point.

LOCATION

There are trigger points all over the body (Figure 2-1). Every muscle has trigger points, whether inactive, active, or latent, and most muscles have more than two trigger points. The location of a trigger point varies depending on an individual's routine, exercise habits, or profession. Trigger point charts (myofascial, neuromuscular, or oriental, to name a few) are available to therapists and show the most common referral areas associated with trigger points. However, because every body is different, the charts do not necessarily represent the *only* referral areas where a trigger point could refer pain. Keep in mind that, like everything in the practice of massage therapy, this is not an exact science and no one person has all the right answers.

A trigger point is an indication of a physiological dysfunction and is the first warning sign that things are not well in the neuromusculoskeletal system. Similar to the "check engine" light in a car, a trigger point is a warning of dysfunction, and if left unchecked could represent very serious consequences. The following is a list of reasons a trigger point might activate, with blank entries for your own thoughts at the end:

1. Contracture in the muscle
2. Increased muscle tonus
3. Constriction and hypersensitivity in the skin in local or referred area
4. Increased pressure in the joints associated with the muscle
5. Decreased activity in visceral organs associated through depressed autonomic nerve activity (especially with spinal subluxations)
6. Constriction in local circulation resulting from hypertonus of and constriction in the muscle
7. Vasoconstriction in referred area from effects in the autonomic nervous system
8. Development of secondary and associated trigger points as a result of compensation from the effects of the primary trigger point
9. Muscle overuse
10. Poor posture
11. Poor ergonomics
12. Overstretch
13. Lack of stretching
14. Incorrect technique when exercising

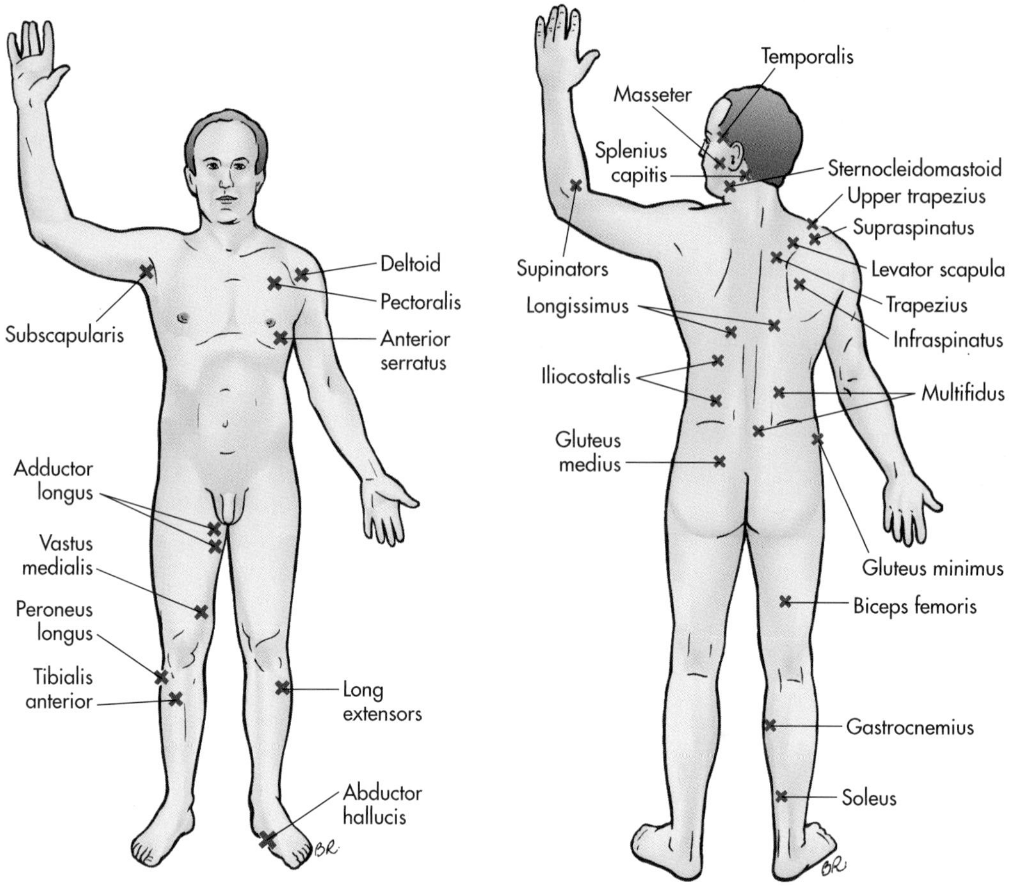

FIGURE 2-1 ■ Common trigger points. (From Fritz S: *Mosby's fundamentals of therapeutic massage,* ed. 3. St. Louis, 2004, Mosby.)

15. Lack of exercise
16. ____________________
17. ____________________
18. ____________________
19. ____________________
20. ____________________

PALPATION

Palpating or finding a trigger point is not easy; students often get frustrated because they usually can only find the trigger point by using a chart and cannot feel it to effectively release it. It takes a lot of practice before a trigger point is felt, not to mention mastering the technique. Therapists often argue about what a trigger point feels like, and they are often misguided. For example, therapists confuse knots with trigger points and proceed to work on the knot with direct finger pressure; unfortunately, this will cause extreme pain to the client and result in failure to effectively treat the nodal point. Some indications of a trigger point are:

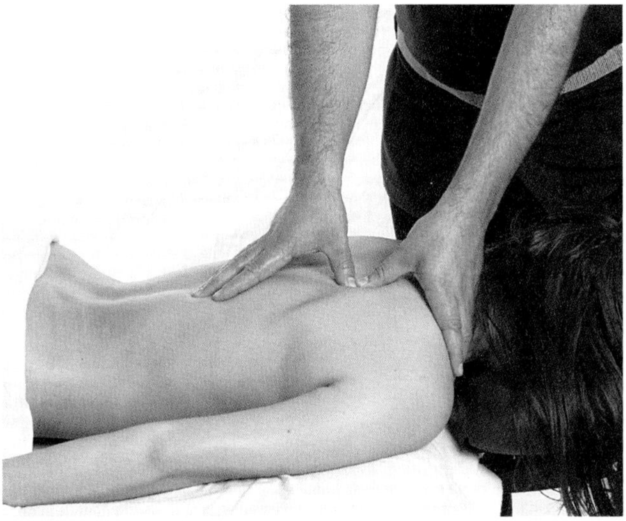

FIGURE 2-2 ■

- Tender spot
- Slight indentation in the muscle
- Ischemic tender point
- Hyperemic tender point
- Warm area on the skin not more than 1 inch in diameter
- Around scar tissue
- Around knots
- Neuromuscular junction

The only way to learn how to effectively palpate a trigger point is to practice using a trigger point chart, keeping in mind that practice makes perfect.

RELEASE METHODS

Ischemic compression is pressure applied by therapist (Figure 2-2).

Typical Treatment Method

1. Treat superficial trigger points first, applying direct pressure over each trigger point for 8 to 20 seconds or until the pain is gone. Notice changes in feel, density, and pain intensity (ask client for feedback using the 1-10 pain tolerance scale detailed later).
2. Communicate with your client and ask if there are any referral patterns or pathways.
3. Apply deep effleurage, petrissage, or friction.
4. If the trigger point did not deactivate, return to the same trigger point and repeat the treatment 3 to 4 times, removing as much of the pain as possible.
5. If the pain intensifies, hold for a few more seconds until it releases or come back to it again later. The key is not to fatigue the trigger point.

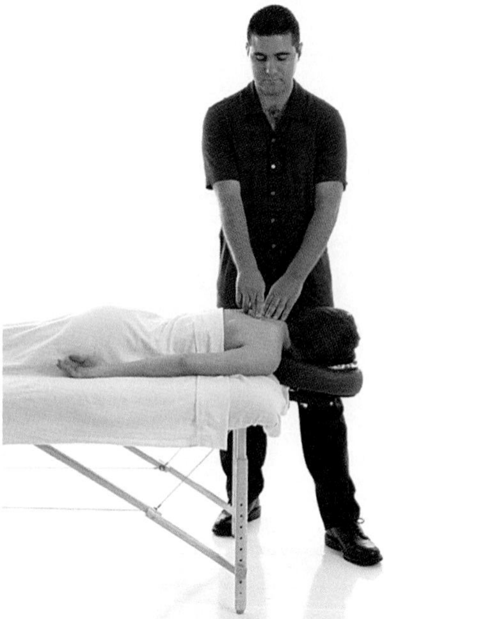

FIGURE 2-3 ■ Apply direct pressure over the trigger point.

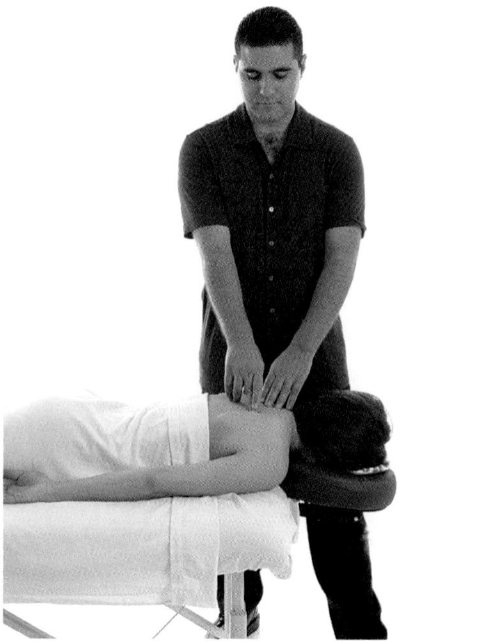

FIGURE 2-4 ■ Apply deep effleurage, pettrisage, or friction.

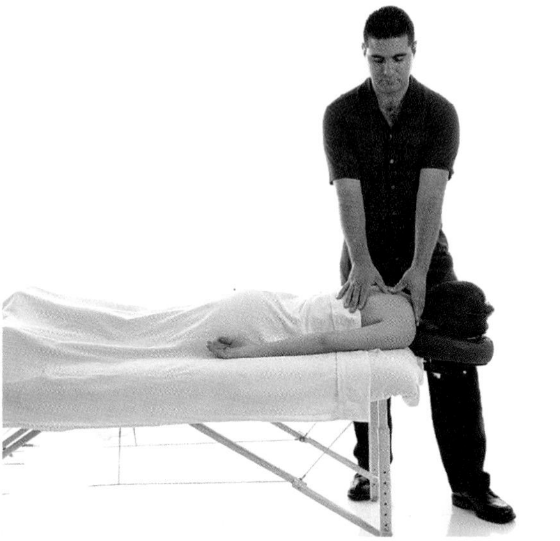

FIGURE 2-5 ■ Return to the same trigger point and repeat treatment 3 to 4 times, removing as much of the pain as possible.

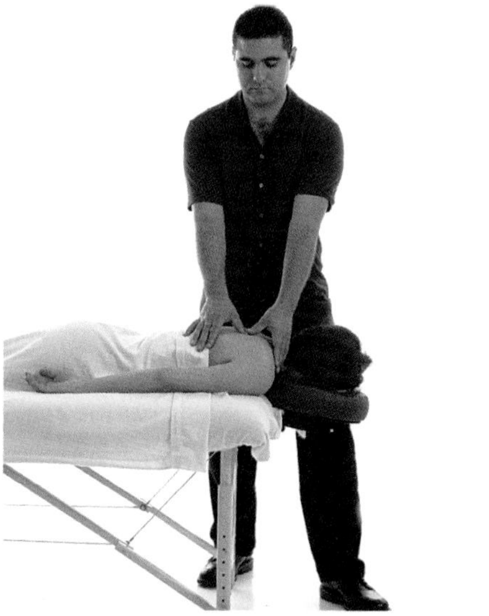

FIGURE 2-6 ■ If the pain intensifies, just hold for a few more seconds until it releases, or come back to it later.

6. You can vary the pressure gradually, moving with the point as it changes and releases; however, keep in mind that the key is to apply equal pressure to the point until it is released (Figures 2-3, 2-4, 2-5, 2-6, 2-7).

Examples of **stretching** include passive, assisted, proprioceptive neuromuscular facilitation (PNF), and developmental (please refer to Chapter 29 for more stretching examples).

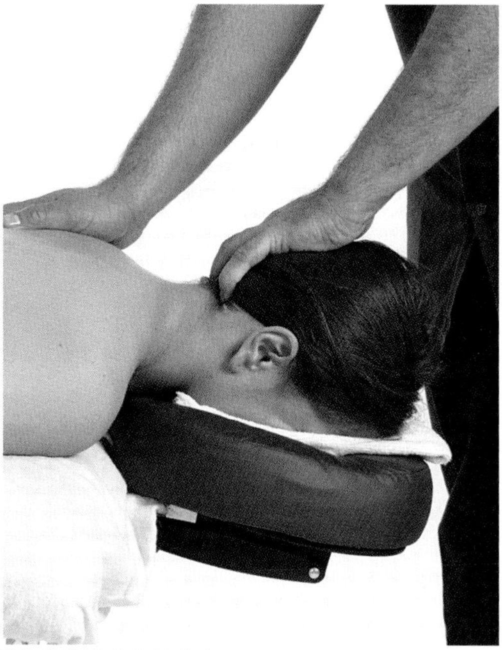

FIGURE 2-7 ■ The key is to apply equal pressure often, until the trigger point is released.

CAUTION

Work within your client's pain tolerance. Contrary to popular belief, the concept "No pain, no gain" must *never* be used in the application of this or any other techniques outlined in this handbook. It is important to remember that all techniques must be applied in accordance with a client's pain-tolerance level. One way to determine this is to use a scale: 1 (slight discomfort) to 10 (extreme pain). It is strongly recommended that a therapist apply all techniques shown in this book only for clients with a pain-tolerance level of 8 or below.

Pressure applied must be deep enough and held long enough to deactivate the trigger point. Most therapists are either afraid or too eager to apply too much pressure. A therapist must never be afraid, or show the client fear, when treating trigger points. At the same time, a therapist must never *under any circumstance* exceed a client's pain tolerance. We should never use the "no pain, no gain" approach to work on anyone; doing so will cause the contrary effect on the muscle.

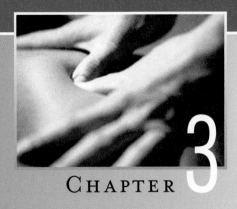

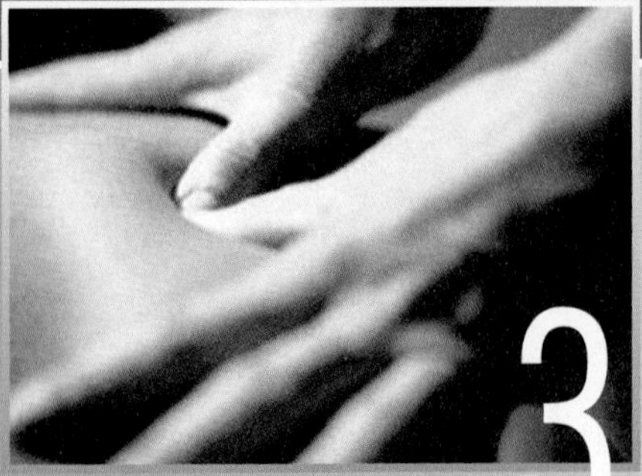

CHAPTER 3

FRICTION

OUTLINE

Friction Definition
Cross-Fiber Friction
Deep Transverse Friction
Circular Friction
Palm Friction
With-Fiber Friction

KEY TERMS

Friction
Range of motion
Cross-fiber friction
Deep transverse friction
Circular friction
Palm friction
With-fiber friction

OBJECTIVES

Upon completion of this chapter the reader will have the information necessary to:

1 **Define friction**
2 **Identify various friction techniques**
3 **Describe and implement common friction techniques to specific body parts**
4 **Classify friction techniques according to the area being treated**

Friction is defined as the application of deep movement with the digits, palm, knuckle, or elbow on a soft tissue in an effort to break up adhesions, scar tissue, or nodules that restrict blood flow, **range of motion** (ROM), movement, or sensation to that area. Friction is intended for soft tissue application and should never be applied directly to a bony landmark.

Most common friction techniques include:

- Cross-fiber friction
- Deep transverse friction
- Circular friction
- Palm friction
- With-fiber friction

CROSS-FIBER FRICTION

Cross-fiber friction is generally applied to the muscle belly, origins, and insertions. As with any other friction technique, cross-fiber friction is correctly applied only when a therapist has a thorough knowledge of the muscular and skeletal system, including muscle origins, insertions, muscle fiber direction, endangerment sites, and bony landmarks (Figure 3-1).

PROCEDURE

The correct application of cross-fiber friction includes *all* of the following (Figures 3-2 and 3-3):

1. Ensure the client is positioned correctly.
2. Determine the muscle to be treated (origin, insertion, and fiber direction).
3. Therapist *must* use correct body posture in relation to the area being treated.

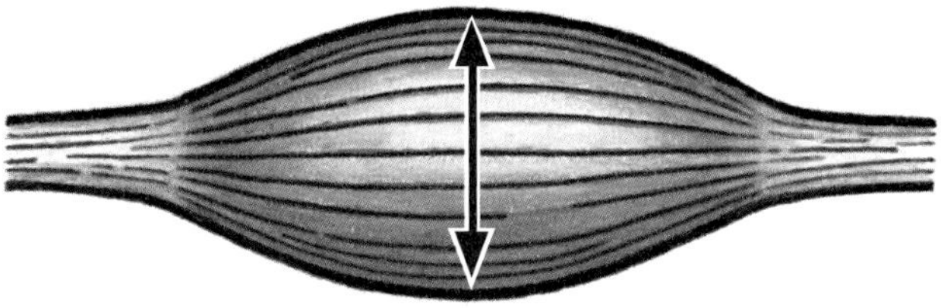

FIGURE 3-1 ■ Cross-fiber friction must be applied perpendicular to muscle fiber direction.

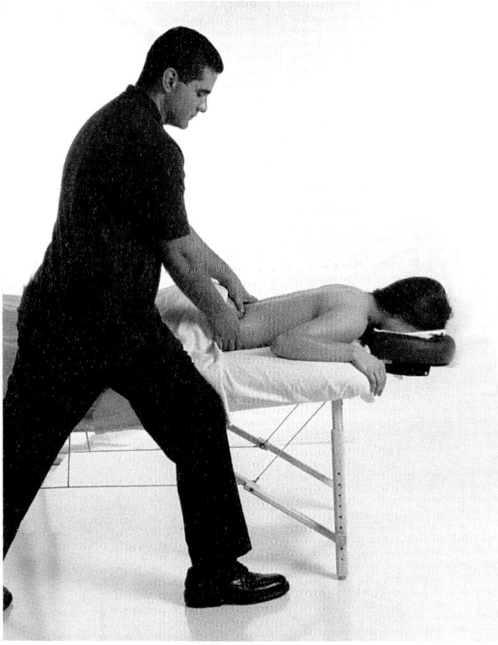

FIGURE 3-2 ■ The therapist MUST use correct body posture in relation to area being treated.

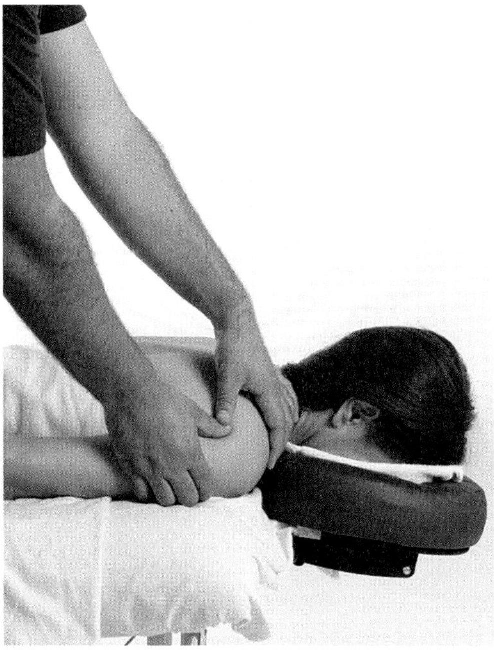

FIGURE 3-3 ■ Technique is applied perpendicular to muscle fiber direction.

4. Proper warm-up technique must be administered.
5. Technique is applied perpendicular to muscle fiber direction and in accordance with client's pain-tolerance level (not to exceed 8 on a 1-10 pain scale).
6. Pressure is gradually increased as client and muscle permits.
7. Proper cool-down techniques are applied.

DEEP TRANSVERSE FRICTION

Popularized by James Cyriax, this method broadens the fibrous tissues of muscles, tendons, or ligaments, breaking down the unwanted fibrous adhesions and thereby restoring mobility to muscles. Although cross-fiber and **deep transverse friction** are popularly believed to be the same, it is this author's opinion that deep transverse friction can be applied at a deeper level than cross-fiber to a muscle grain, incorporating muscle movement at times, e.g., rotating the forearm at the time of technique application on the extensors of the hand.

Deep transverse friction can also be applied to create a controlled re-injury of the tissue, which results in:

1. Restructuring of the connective tissue.
2. Increased circulation.
3. Temporary analgesia.
4. Increased ROM.

PROCEDURE (Figures 3-4 and 3-5)

1. Find the area to be treated.
2. Explain to the client that deep friction can be painful; however, you will be using the 1-10 scale to gauge pain level.

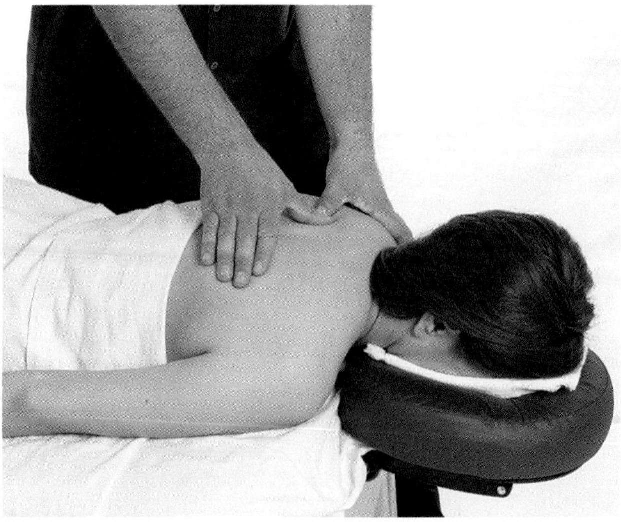

FIGURE 3-4 ■ Position client using the appropriate positioning technique.

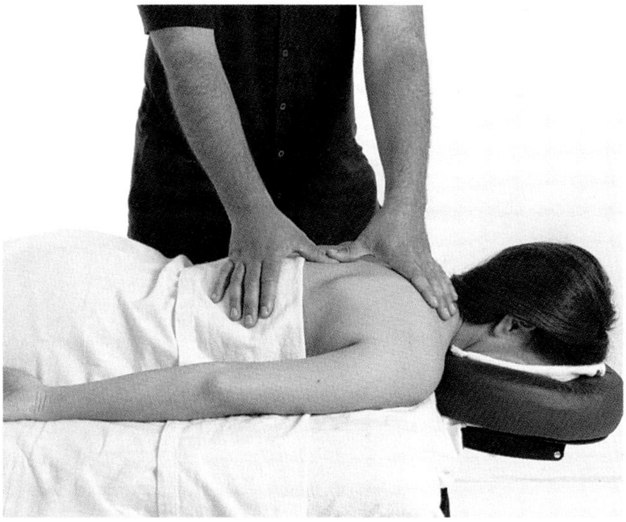

FIGURE 3-5 ■ Friction must be given with sufficient sweep (depth) and a back and forth motion.

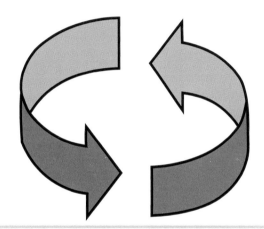

FIGURE 3-6 ■ Circular friction.

3. Position the client using the appropriate positioning technique.
4. Friction must be given with sufficient sweep (depth) and a back and forth motion.

CIRCULAR FRICTION

Circular friction is often used in an effort to increase hyperemia in an area and is often applied around bony landmarks, such as joints or the infraspinus fossa. It can also be used in the treatment of ligaments to increase synovial fluid secretion and aid in breaking up localized adhesions. This technique should be applied using a circular, controlled digital movement. Care should be taken to avoid performing friction directly on a bone (Figure 3-6).

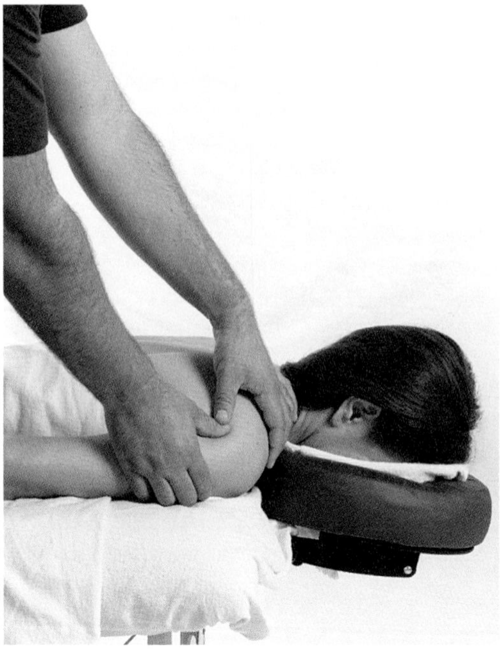

FIGURE 3-7 ■

PROCEDURE (Figure 3-7)

1. Ensure the client is positioned correctly.
2. Determine the area to be treated (joint composition).
3. Ensure the joint has proper support.
4. Therapist *must* use correct body posture in relation to the area being treated.
5. Proper warm-up technique must be administered.
6. Technique should be applied in accordance with the client's pain-tolerance level (not to exceed 8 on a 1-10 pain scale).
7. Pressure is gradually increased as client and muscle permits.
8. Proper cool-down techniques are applied.

PALM FRICTION

Palm friction can be applied with one or two hands and is not intended to be applied as deeply as deep transverse friction. This technique is typically used on large muscle areas (e.g., quadriceps, latissimus dorsi, or trapezius) to increase circulation to a large area, break up superficial adhesions, increase blood flow, and increase tissue pliability.

PROCEDURE (Figure 3-8)

1. Ensure the client is positioned correctly.
2. Determine the area to be treated (muscles involved).
3. Therapist *must* use correct body posture in relation to the area being treated.
4. Proper warm-up technique must be administered.

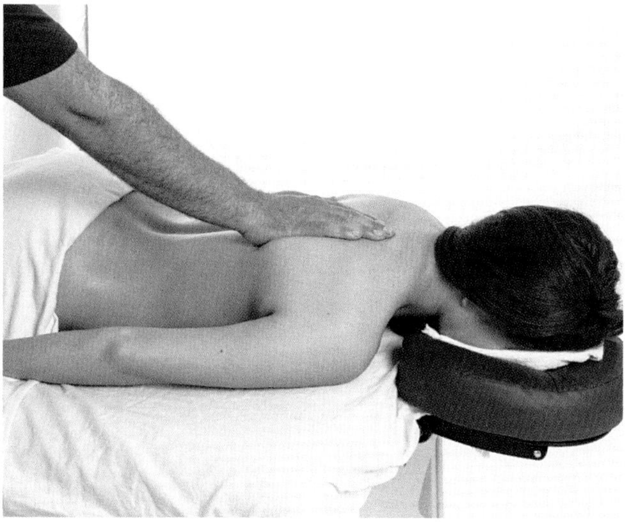

FIGURE 3-8 ■

5. Technique is applied, avoiding bony landmarks, in accordance with client's pain-tolerance level (not to exceed 8 on a 1-10 pain scale).
6. Pressure is gradually increased as client and muscle permits.
7. Proper cool-down techniques are applied.

WITH-FIBER FRICTION (SPREADING)

With-fiber friction, also known as stripping or spreading, is generally applied to the length of the muscle. Aside from increasing circulation, breaking up scar tissue, and realigning muscle fibers, this technique is commonly used to treat nodules (knots). In an effort to treat knots, therapists often mistakenly use techniques such as cross-fiber, circular friction, and direct pressure; however, these techniques only aggravate and increase pain to the area. To understand the reasoning behind the benefit of using with-fiber friction, nodule composition must be understood.

A knot is a combination of spastic and intertwined muscle fibers. Although knots can appear in any area of the body, they are most commonly encountered on the shoulders, back, thighs, legs, and feet. To successfully treat a knot, muscle fibers must be realigned according to their original direction. Therefore strokes should start on the knot and be directed away from the area, as shown below. Additionally this will assist sensory nerves to not activate, which can cause a muscle to spasm when an incorrect technique is applied (Figure 3-9).

PROCEDURE (Figure 3-10)

1. Ensure the client is positioned correctly.
2. Determine the area to be treated (muscles involved).
3. Therapist *must* use correct body posture in relation to the area being treated.
4. Proper warm-up technique must be administered.

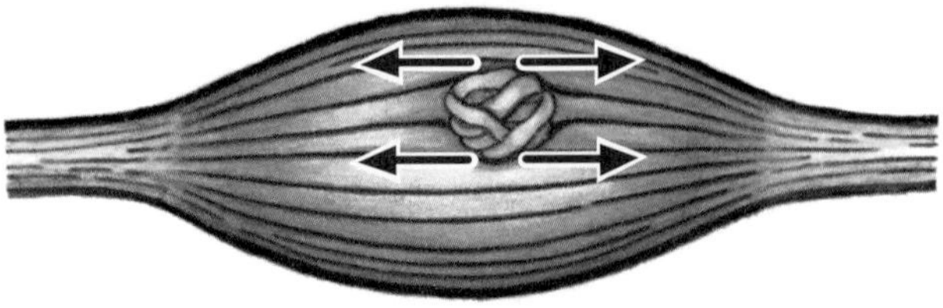

FIGURE 3-9 ■ With-fiber friction.

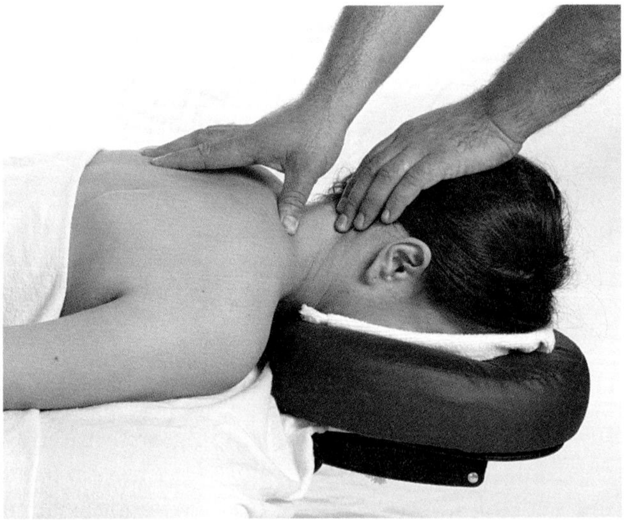

FIGURE 3-10 ■

5. Technique is applied away from nodule, avoiding bony landmarks, in accordance with client's pain-tolerance level (not to exceed 8 on a 1-10 pain scale).
6. Pressure is gradually increased as client and muscle permits.
7. Proper cool-down techniques are applied.

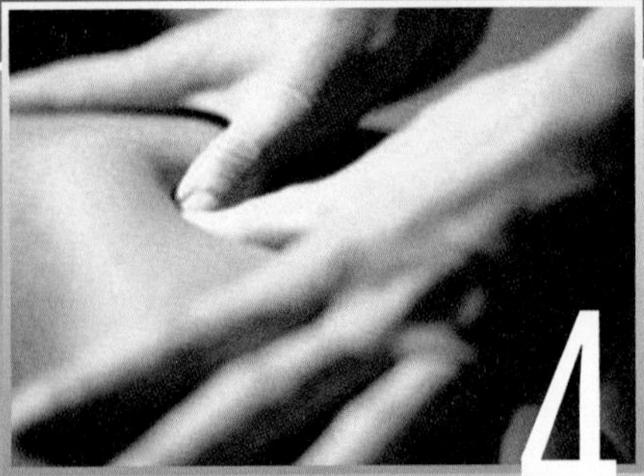

CHAPTER 4

MYOFASCIAL RELEASE

OUTLINE

Myofascial Dysfunction Definition
Facts about the Fascia
Treatment
Contraindications
Deep Tissue Sculpting

KEY TERMS

Myofascial release
Fascia

OBJECTIVES

Upon completion of this chapter the reader will have the information necessary to:

1 **Identify Myofascial Release (MFR)**
2 **Identify various MFR techniques**
3 **Describe and perform common MFR techniques**
4 **Become proficient in various common muscle specific MFR techniques**
5 **List common MFR contraindications**

Myofascial dysfunction is an abnormal fascia condition that causes the development of poor posture or structural misalignment and could result in the displacement of bones or the entrapment of blood vessels and nerves.

Myofascial release (MFR) is known as a deep tissue technique that addresses the **fascia** and surrounding tissue that connects all muscles, bones, and internal organs. There are various techniques attributed with MFR, but for practical purposes we will discuss deep tissue sculpting.

FACTS ABOUT THE HEALTHY FASCIA

1. Resembles a plastic wrapping but has the consistency of the filmy, slippery tissue
2. Provides the body with strength, support, elasticity, and cushion
3. Protects the organs and provides contour to the limbs

4. Provides a covering that helps conserve body heat
5. Is well hydrated, pliable, and moves freely

TREATMENT

Myofascial release is a technique that is best performed slowly and patiently. The main goal is to increase tissue pliability in an effort to enhance blood flow between tissues. It does not require the use of lotion or cream (friction is desired to aid in release) and is performed slowly and patiently. Compressions are directional, and angles of treatment are determined by the structure of the tissue, e.g., the therapist should check tissue pliability in all angles before determining in which direction the restriction is occurring (Figures 4-1 through 4-4). This method can also be performed on clients who are clothed.

MFR techniques include:

- Softening
- Lengthening
- Broadening
- Separating the fascia

CONTRAINDICATIONS

1. Malignancies
2. Aneurysm
3. Acute rheumatoid arthritis

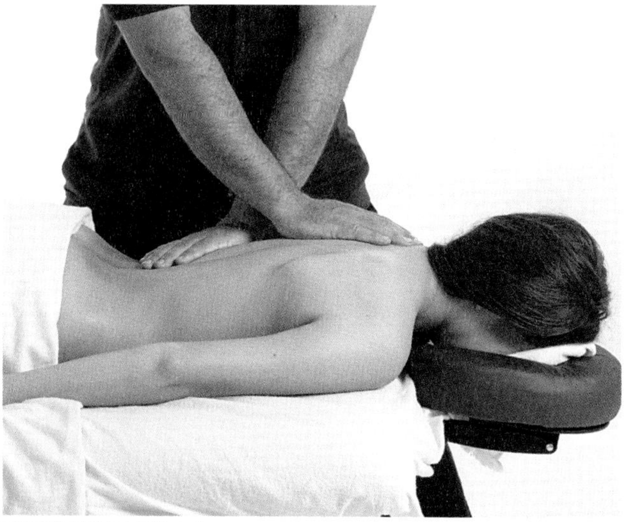

FIGURE 4-1 ■ Softening.

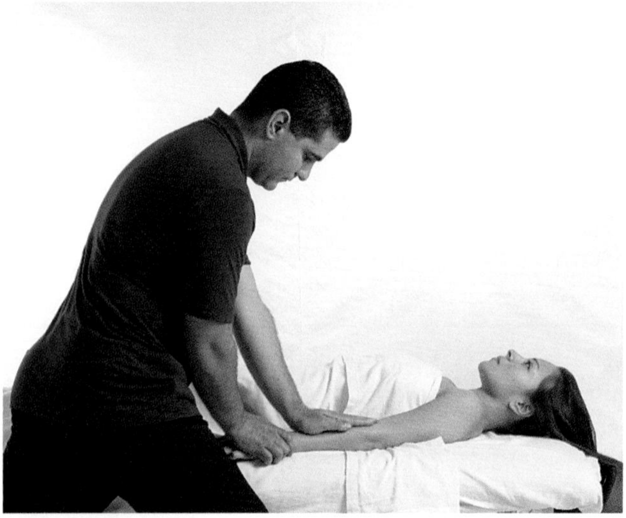

FIGURE 4-2 ■ Lengthening.

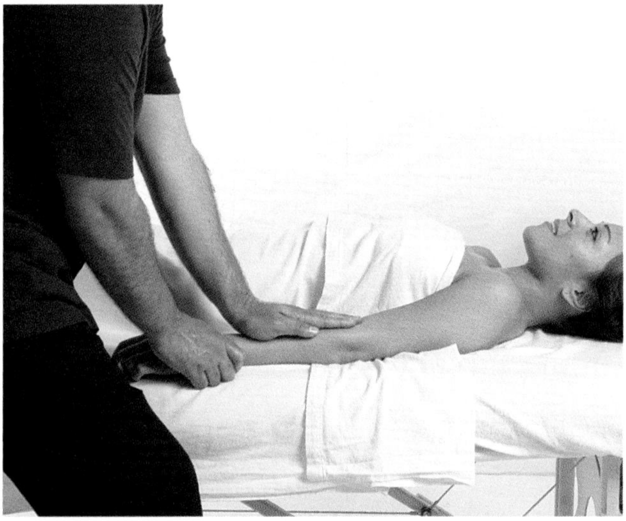

FIGURE 4-3 ■ Broadening.

4. Open wounds
5. Serious bruises
6. Fractures
7. Brittle bones
8. Skin irritations

DEEP TISSUE SCULPTING

BACK AND PECTORAL GIRDLE

Objective: Elongate the extensor muscles of the back and release pectoral girdle.

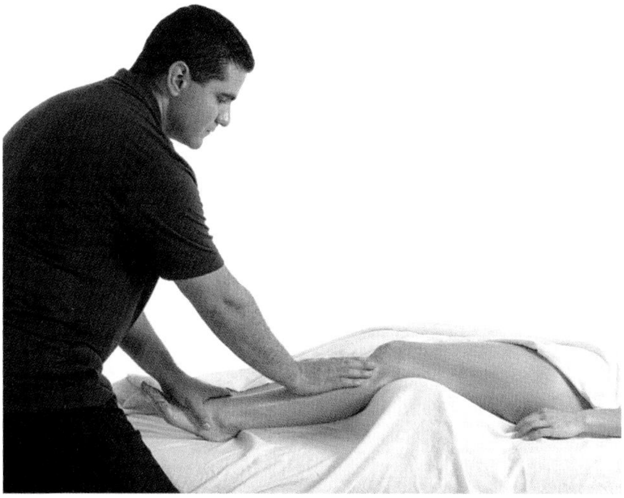

FIGURE 4-4 ■ Separating the fascia.

Position: Client is prone with proper placement of bolsters/pillows under ankles and anterior superior iliac spine (ASIS) if needed (e.g., if the client has lordosis [see Chapter 18]).

UPPER TRAPEZIUS

Objective: Elongate the upper trapezius fibers across the shoulders in an effort to release and broaden the shoulder muscles.

Procedure: Compress and/or stroke the trapezius from near the neck to the acromioclavicular joint. Compress and/or stroke along the superior edge of the spine of the scapula, moving laterally out of the acromioclavicular joint.

Hint: Do not use very deep compression.

LOWER TRAPEZIUS

Objective: Elongate the lower trapezius fibers and release the scapula to a more balanced position.

Procedure: Sculpt along the upper vertebral border of the scapula and continue downward at an angle toward T12.

Hint: Do not use very deep compression. You may use multidirectional sculpting of the trapezius, rhomboid major, erector spinae, and latissimus dorsi.

TERES MAJOR AND MINOR

Objective: Release the teres muscles.

Procedure:

1. Release teres muscle attachments along the lateral border of the scapula with compressions beginning near the inferior angle.
2. Release bellies of the two with compression into the V formed by the teres minor and the deltoid.
3. Release teres minor insertion by compressing under the deltoid to the greater tubercle of the humerus.

RHOMBOIDS

Objective: To elongate and release rhomboids to allow the scapula to assume a balanced position.

Procedure:

1. Begin stroking/compressing the rhomboids from C7 toward the insertion (vertebral border of the scapula).
2. Continue with a series of stroking and compressions to the remainder of the rhomboid muscles.

SPINE AND ILIAC CREST AREA

Objective: To elongate and release muscles and fascia attaching to the spine (trapezius, rhomboids, and erector spinae).

Procedure: From a position in front of the client's head, begin stroking/compressing the muscles on each side of the spine, starting from C7 to the sacrum. Work either both sides simultaneously or one at a time (right then left).

Precautions: Do not stroke or place any pressure directly over the spinous process.

VERTEBRAE

Objective: To release the muscles and fascia attaching along the spinous process of the vertebrae.

Procedure: Using a narrow tool (T-bar, thumb, or other digit), compress against the side of the spinous process (light to medium pressure) of each vertebra from C7 down to sacrum.

ILIAC CREST AREA

Objective: To release tension in the muscles attaching onto the iliac crest.

Procedure: Compress superiorly to the iliac crest; begin near the sacroiliac joint and progress laterally, making a series of compression and/or sculpting.

LOWER EXTREMITIES AND LOWER TRUNK

Objective: To elongate the extensor muscles of the trunk that connects the torso and legs.

Position: Client is prone with proper placement of bolsters/pillows under ankles and ASIS if needed (e.g., if the client has lordosis).

Assessment:

- Excessive interiorly convex curvature of the lumbar spine (lordosis).
- Excessive anterior or posterior angles of the pelvis (compare ASIS and posterior superior iliac spine [PSIS]).
- Flattened lumbar curvature.
- Uneven height between right and left iliac crest.

Tightness: Erector spinae, abdominals, iliopsoas, quadratus lumborum, 6 deep lateral rotators of the hip, hamstrings, and quadriceps muscles.

DEFINING THE SACRUM AND RELEASING GLUTEUS MAXIMUS

Objective: To elongate the gluteus maximus.

Procedure:

1. Compress along the border of the sacrum.
2. Make a series of compressions, moving inferiorly along the sacrum.
3. Compress and/or stroke the gluteus maximus from the origin toward the insertion into the iliotibial tract, elongating and sculpting the fascia.

Precautions:

- The sciatic nerve is embedded beneath the gluteus maximus and may be sensitive to deep compressions. Change position, direction, and depth of pressure if the client feels an electrical, burning, numbing, or painful sensation down the posterior leg.
- Be sensitive to the client's needs near the coccyx.

LENGTHENING OF THE HAMSTRING GROUP (SEMI-TENDINOSUS, SEMI-MEMBRANOSUS, BICEPS FEMORIS)

Objective: To elongate the hamstring muscle group and release the ischial tuberosity.

Procedure:

1. Begin with compression on the ischial tuberosity with the heel of the palm or the fist.
2. Continue with compression or slow sculpting stroke down the whole hamstring muscle group to a few inches above the knee.
3. Finish with sculpting on this muscle group attachment on the tibia and fibula.

Precautions: Remember that varicose veins are contraindication to massage.

RELEASE OF THE QUADRICEPS GROUP (RECTUS FEMORIS, VASTUS LATERALIS, VASTUS MEDIALIS, VASTUS INTERMEDIUS)

Objective: To elongate the quadriceps muscle group and release the ASIS.

Position: Client is in the supine position.

Procedure:

1. Begin with compressing the origin of the rectus femoris just below the ASIS.
2. Follow with the release of the muscle down toward the knee or make a series of compressions to just above the knee.
3. Use a smaller tool (T-bar) to sculpt the attachments of the quadriceps at each side of the patella.

ABDOMINAL RELEASE

Objective: To release tension in the rectus, oblique, and transversus abdominis muscles.

Position: Client is in the supine position.

Procedure:

1. Very gently use the heel of the hand to compress gently into the abdominal muscles.

2. Make a series of compressions to release the entire abdomen.
3. Compress from near the xiphoid process along the inferior edge of the ribcage.

Precautions:

- Proceed slowly to avoid painful pressure on the abdominal group.
- Do not use this procedure on clients who are pregnant, menstruating, or have abdominal pain.
- Avoid painful pressure on rib 11 (floating rib) by ending the ribcage compressions at the end of the costal cartilage.

ANTERIOR FLAT OF THE ILIUM

Objective: To increase awareness of the pelvis, abdominal muscles and iliopsoas muscle.

Position: Client is in the supine position.

Procedure:

1. Begin near the ASIS and perform gentle compressions toward the pubic ramus.
2. Sculpt slowly and gently down the slope of the ilium.

Precautions:

- Keep the anterior side of the fingers against the flat of the ilium.
- Do not apply direct pressure inferiorly to the inguinal ligament.

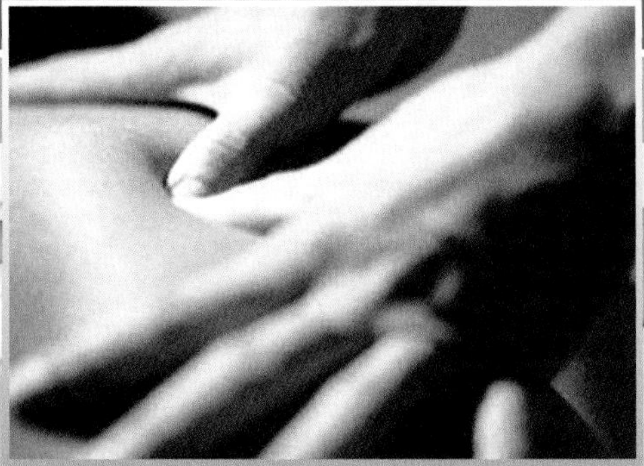
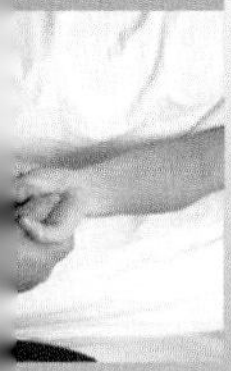
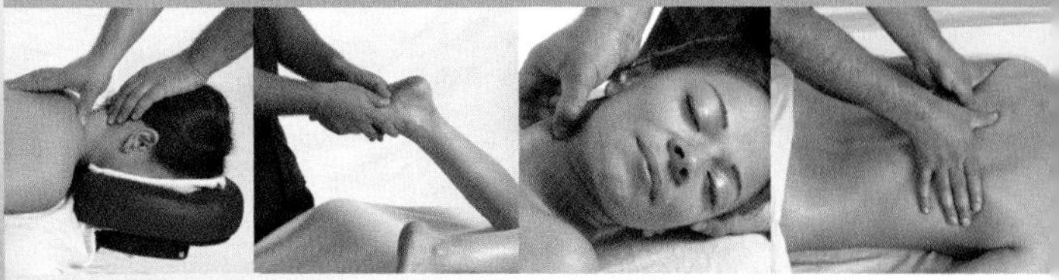

PART TWO

TREATMENT ROUTINES

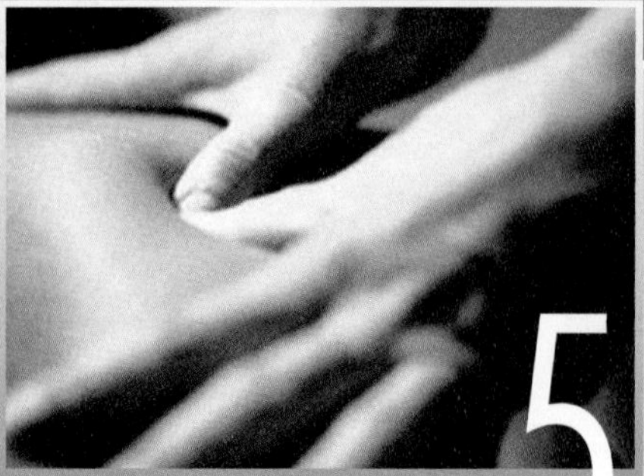

CHAPTER 5

NECK PAIN AND HEADACHE

OUTLINE

Definition and symptoms
Indications
Contraindications
Neck pain and headache routine

KEY TERM

Headache

OBJECTIVES

Upon completion of this chapter the reader will have the information necessary to:

1. **Define common neck pain and headache causes**
2. **Describe common headache symptoms**
3. **Identify common routine indications**
4. **Classify common routine contraindications**
5. **Understand and perform a neck pain and headache routine**

DEFINITION AND SYMPTOMS

Neck pain and **headaches** can be caused by trauma, injury, stress, poor sleeping pattern or position, prolonged use of a computer, poor ergonomics, poor posture, a trapped nerve caused by a bulge in one of the discs between the vertebrae, or arthritis of the neck. Pain can range from very mild to a severe, burning feeling. If untreated, it can quickly develop from acute (sudden and intense, i.e., crick in the neck, facet syndrome, spasms, or muscular rheumatism) to chronic.

⚠ Icon represents an area where extreme caution should be used to avoid damage or compression to underlying or neighboring vessels.

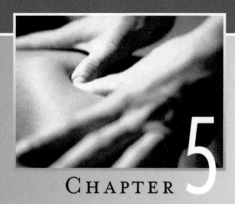

Indications

- Torticollis
- Whiplash (see Chapter 10)
- Neck stiffness
- Limited range of motion (ROM)

Contraindications

- Edema
- Severe cervical herniations
- Acute trauma (accident 0-36 hours before the onset of pain)
- Peripheral vascular disease (PVD)

NECK PAIN AND HEADACHE ROUTINE

POSITION: CLIENT IS SUPINE

PROCEDURE:

1 Regulate your client's breathing by placing one hand over the diaphragm and the other over the abdomen and performing a gentle rocking motion.
2 Initiate the massage by spreading lotion, with effleurage strokes, over the upper pectoralis major area, shoulders, upper trapezius, and posterior neck region.
3 Effleurage the posterior neck area from the superior angle of the scapula up to the occipital ridge (base of the neck).
4 Gently place neck (head in neutral position) onto overlapped hands and perform a gentle side to side rocking motion.
5 Rotate head to the left and effleurage the right side of the neck using long strokes that begin at the shoulders and move up toward the occipital ridge.
6 Petrissage in a V shape the same side, being careful not to compress the underlying artery with the thumb (reposition hand if pulse is felt) (Figure 5-1).

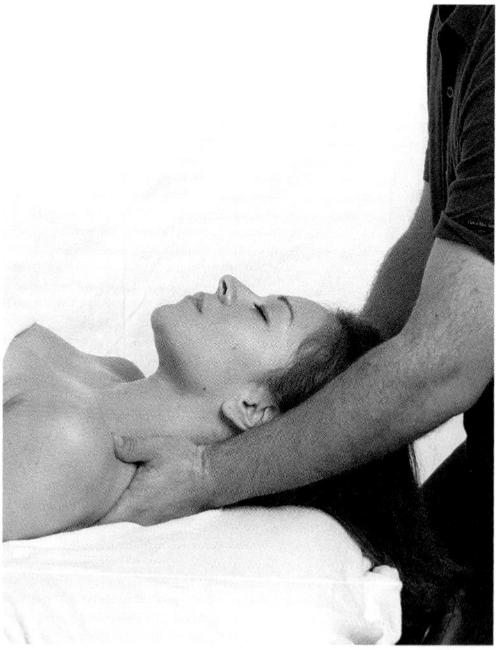

FIGURE 5-1

7 Return neck to neutral position and gently rock neck with overlapped hands (Figure 5-2).

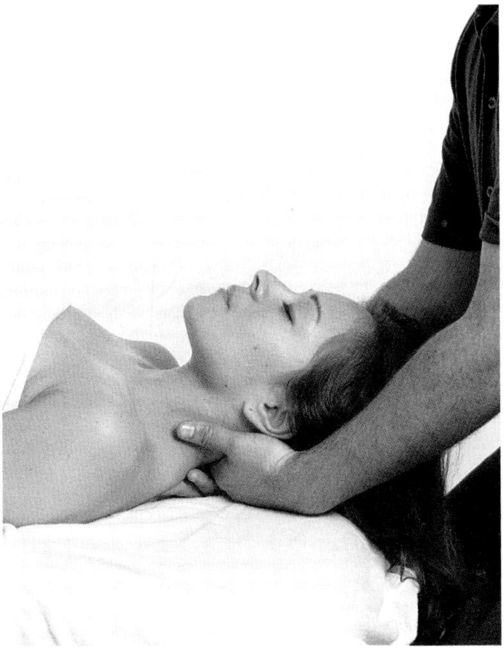

FIGURE 5-2 ■

8 Effleurage posterior neck several times by placing hand under C7 and moving up toward the occipital ridge.
9 Repeat steps 5 through 8 to the left side of the neck.
10 Perform with-fiber friction with the thumb to the posterior cervical muscles beginning at the occipital ridge and ending at the base of the shoulders.
11 Work only on active trigger points; perform trigger point therapy to the occipital ridge area (Figure 5-3).

NECK PAIN AND HEADACHE ROUTINE

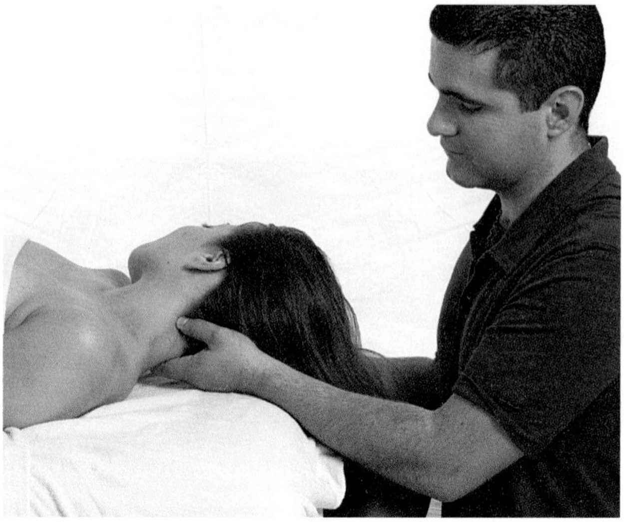

FIGURE 5-3

12 Work only on active trigger points; perform trigger point therapy to the base of the neck (where neck meets shoulder).
13 Effleurage the entire area three times.
14 Perform thumb with-fiber friction to the levator scapulae from superior to inferior (Figure 5-4).

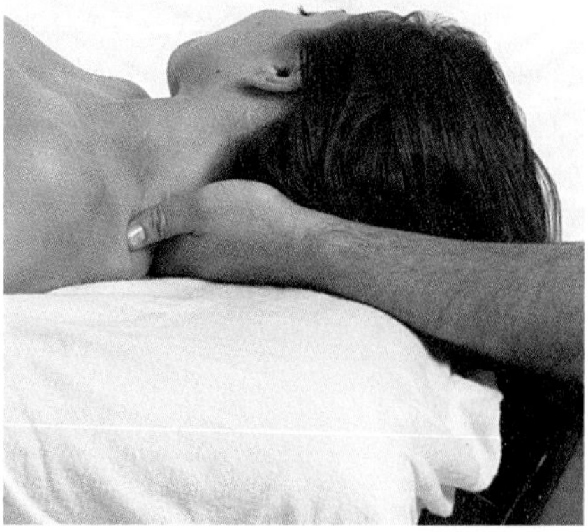

FIGURE 5-4

NECK PAIN AND HEADACHE ROUTINE

15 Massage the temporal muscles by performing circular motions with fingers starting at the scalp and moving down towards the masseter (Figure 5-5).

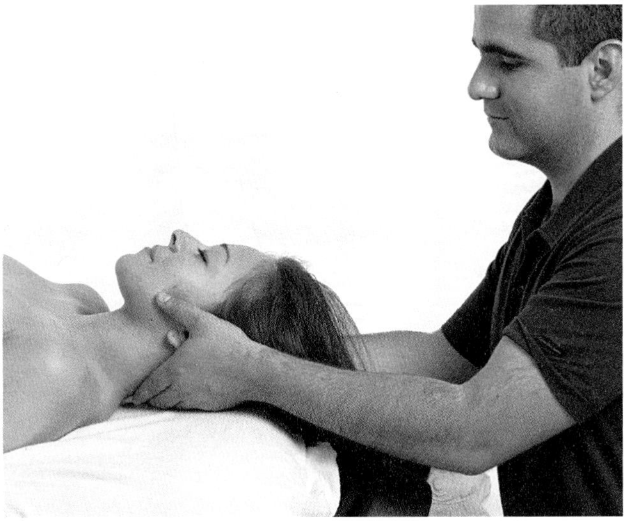

FIGURE 5-5

16 Apply thumb pressure to the midline of the forehead, moving all the way to the temples three times.
17 Finish with feather stroke across the jaw line.

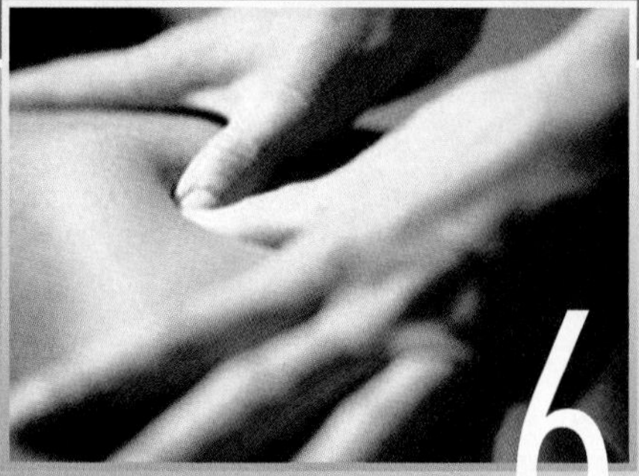

CHAPTER 6

MIGRAINE

OUTLINE

Definition and symptoms
Indications
Contraindications
Migraine routine

KEY TERMS

Migraine

OBJECTIVES

Upon completion of this chapter the reader will have the information necessary to:

1. **Define common migraine causes**
2. **Describe common migraine symptoms**
3. **Identify common migraine routine indications**
4. **Classify common migraine routine contraindications**
5. **Understand and perform a migraine routine**

DEFINITION AND SYMPTOMS

A **migraine** is a headache that is usually very intense and disabling. Migraine headaches can be neurological, neuromuscular, vascular, or nutritional in nature. The word *migraine* originates from the Greek word *hemikranion* (pain affecting one side of the head).

It is estimated that 45 million Americans suffer from chronic headaches, and of those, more than half have migraines. It is also estimated that migraine headaches, particularly ones that affect vision, are a risk factor for stroke in young people.

Characteristics of migraines include attacks of sharp pain that usually involve one half of the cranium and are accompanied by nausea, vomiting, photophobia, and sometimes visual disturbances known as "aura." In some

⚠ Icon represents an area where extreme caution should be used to avoid damage or compression to underlying or neighboring vessels.

patients the incidence of migraine can be reduced through diet changes, by avoiding certain chemicals present in foods such as cheddar cheese, chocolate, and most alcoholic beverages. Other triggers may be stress-related and can be avoided through changes in lifestyle.

Indications

The most common treatments for migraine involve pain pills, injections, changes in lifestyle and diet, deep tissue treatments, exercise, and nontraditional methods such as acupuncture. A client should always check with his or her physician for the appropriate treatment geared to a specific type of headache. The treatment included in this chapter is meant to help individuals with neuromuscular- and postural-related migraines.

Contraindications

- Vascular disorders
- Dietary migraines
- Heart conditions
- Advanced diabetes
- History of stroke
- Vascular migraines

MIGRAINE ROUTINE

POSITION: CLIENT IS IN THE SUPINE POSITION

PROCEDURE:

1 Effleurage the shoulders and posterior neck muscles.
2 Petrissage the client's posterior neck muscles (lightly lubricated), concentrating on the upper trapezius (massage both sides).
3 Hold the head with one hand and thumb-strip next to the lamina groove using the other hand (Figure 6-1).

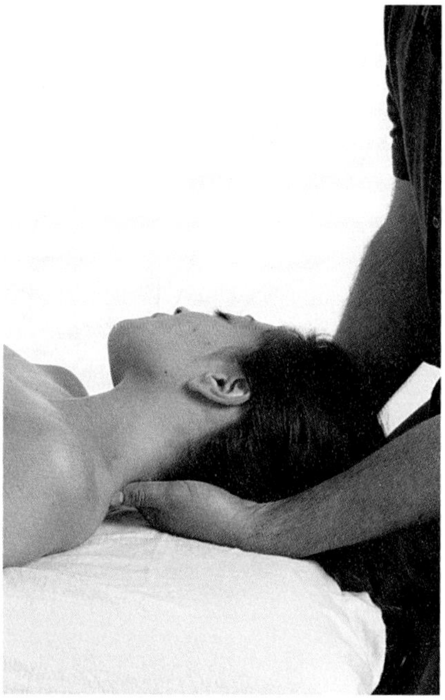

FIGURE 6-1 ■

4 Add side-to-side movement of the head while stripping the muscles.
5 Apply cross-fiber friction and with-fiber friction to the occipital ridge (Figures 6-2 and 6-3).

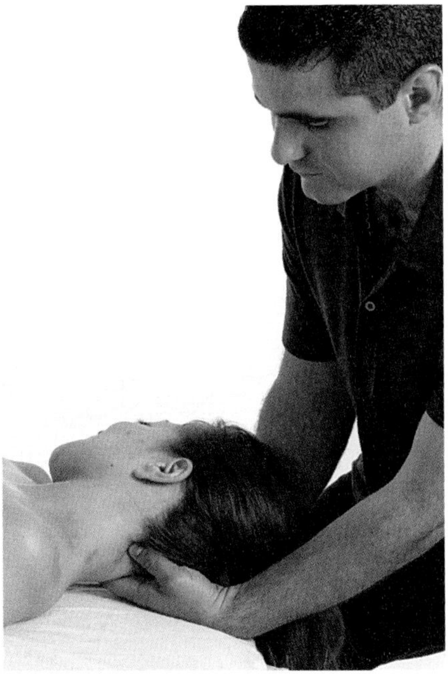

FIGURE 6-2 ■ Add side-to-side movement of the head while stripping the muscles.

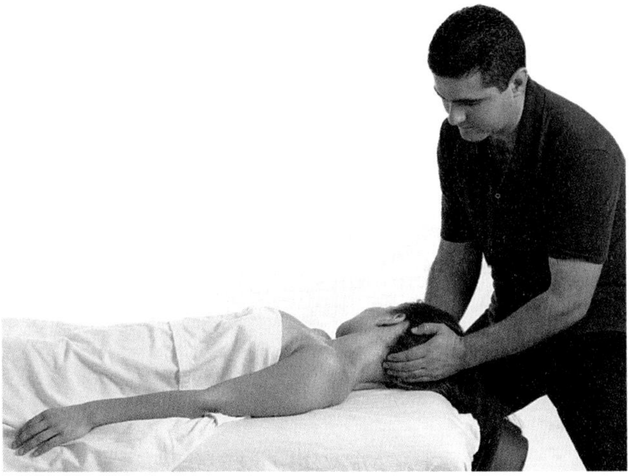

FIGURE 6-3 ■ Apply cross-fiber friction and with-fiber friction to the occipital ridge.

6 Perform occipital release (manual head traction) and hold for 15 to 20 seconds.
7 Use gentle hair-pulling to release the fascia on the head. Run fingers through the hair, grab with a closed fist, and pull. Wait for 5 seconds then twist hand for an additional 5 seconds. Use this technique mainly in the temporalis and parietal areas.
8 Repeat step 5 bilaterally.
9 Pincer-grip the levator scapula and apply thumb stripping (perform technique to both sides) (Figure 6-4).

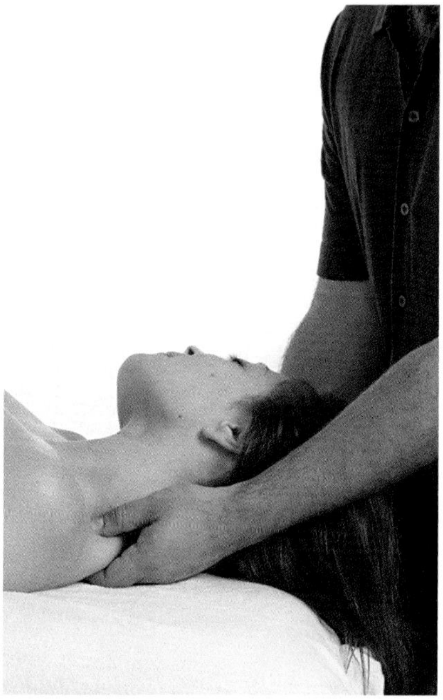

FIGURE 6-4

10 Turn client's head to one side, locate the sternocleidomastoid muscle (SCM) and lightly lubricate (have client lift head to assist in finding muscle).
11 Thumb-strip the SCM from insertion to origin.
12 Apply pincer grip and friction by performing the **money sign** (Figure 6-5).

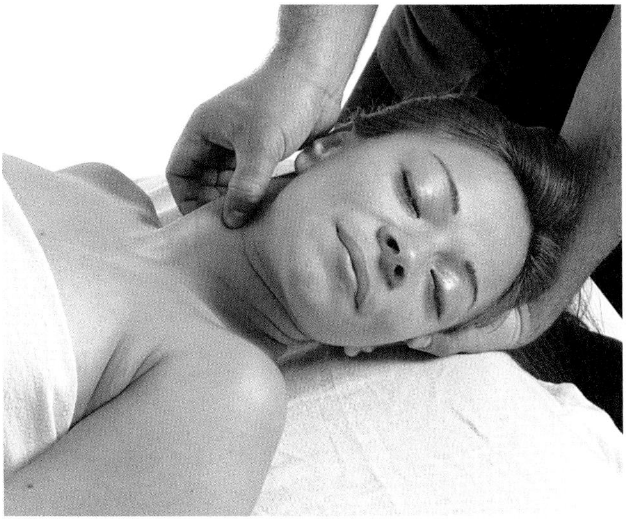

FIGURE 6-5

13 Cross-fiber friction the origin and insertion of the SCM. At clavicular head make sure to friction under the clavicle only after patient exhales.
14 Repeat on the other SCM.

NOTE: If headache persists, make sure to treat the infrahyoid, suprahyoid, and platysma muscles.

MIGRAINE ROUTINE

15 Apply light friction with the gem of the fingers on the inferior portion of the mandible.

16 Have patient swallow several times to locate the trachea.

17 Find and apply gentle superficial gliding lateral to the trachea (Figure 6-6).

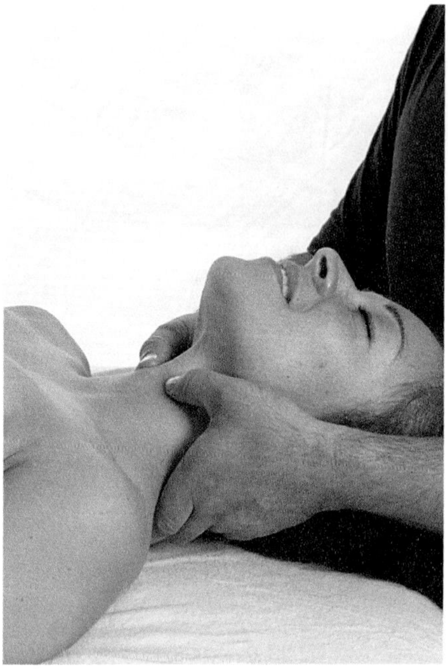

FIGURE 6-6

18 *Slowly* displace the trachea (move to one side) and hold. Friction the muscles of the anterior cervical with the other hand (friction can occur either with the thumb or the other fingers) (Figures 6-7 and 6-8).

⚠ Steps 15 through 18 should be performed with extreme caution, being careful not to damage or compress endangerment vessels.

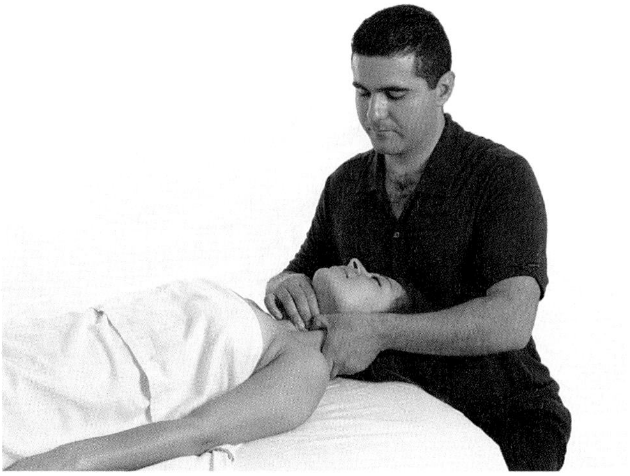

FIGURE 6-7 ■ SLOWLY displace the trachea (move to one side) and hold.

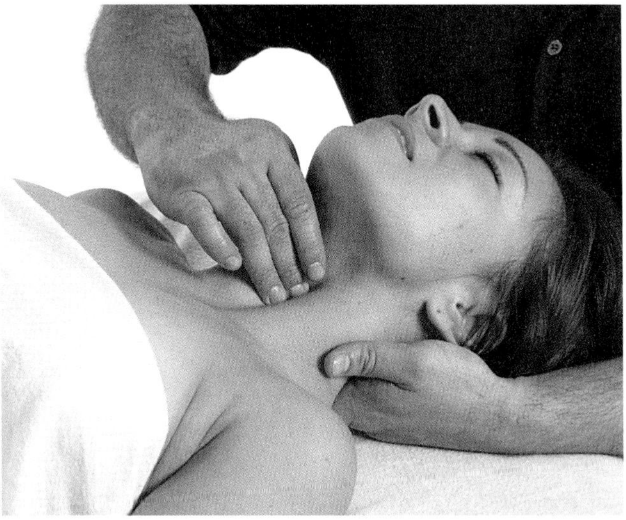

FIGURE 6-8 ■ Friction muscles of the anterior cervical with the other hand.

19 Complete treatment with effleurage and additional hair-pulling if so desired.

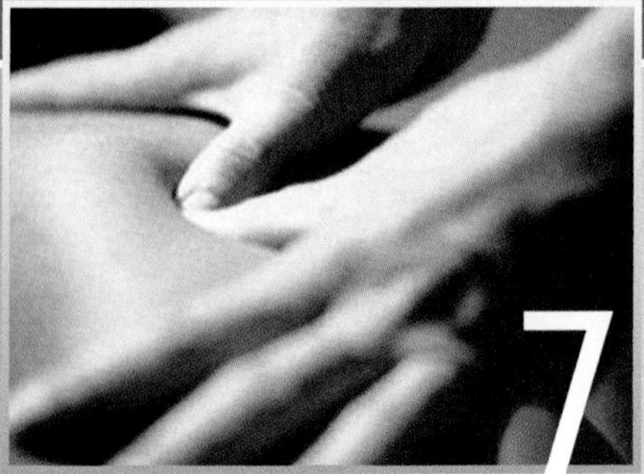

CHAPTER 7

TEMPORAL MANDIBULAR JOINT DISORDER (TMJD)

OUTLINE

Definition and symptoms
Indications
Contraindications
Temporal mandibular joint disorder routine

KEY TERM

Temporal mandibular joint disorder

OBJECTIVES

Upon completion of this chapter the reader will have the information necessary to:

1 **Define common temporal mandibular joint disorder causes**
2 **Describe common temporal mandibular joint disorder symptoms**
3 **Identify common temporal mandibular joint disorder routine indications**
4 **Classify common temporal mandibular joint disorder routine contraindications**
5 **Understand and perform a temporal mandibular joint disorder routine**

DEFINITION AND SYMPTOMS

Temporal mandibular joint disorder results when the muscles of mastication and the jaw joint, or temporal mandibular joint (TMJ), are not working together correctly. It is often masked by headaches, migraines, earaches, tenderness of the jaw muscles, or aching facial pain. Further causes can involve accidents such as injuries to the jaw, head, or neck, or diseases such as arthritis. However, factors relating to the teeth and bite, such as teeth grinding and teeth fit, are believed to be common causes of TMJ disorders. In many cases, if they are treated early, TMJ disorders can be dramatically reduced.

Please refer to the DVD for exact visual technique application of this routine.

Some of the most common symptoms of TMJ disorders include:

- Tenderness of the jaw muscles
- Clicking/popping noises when opening or closing the mouth
- Difficulty opening mouth
- Lock jaw
- Pain brought on by yawning, chewing, or opening the mouth widely
- Certain types of headaches or neck aches
- Pain in or around the ear often spreading to the face

Indications

Because this condition can involve the teeth, chewing muscles, and/or the temporal mandibular joint, treatments vary. Often dentists or physicians will determine a treatment method through a series of phases such as deep tissue treatments, bite adjustments, chewing habit modifications, and in certain cases of severely degenerated joints, surgery might be considered.

The key elements for deep massage treatments are to:

- Eliminate muscle spasms
- Provide relaxation to the muscles of mastication
- Release the pterygoid muscles
- Reduce TMJ disorder

Contraindications

- TMJ disorders resulting from teeth growth patterns
- Open lesions
- Jaw wires
- Severe facial acne

TEMPORAL MANDIBULAR JOINT ROUTINE

POSITION: CLIENT IS STANDING

PROCEDURE:

1 Observe the patient opening and closing his or her jaw. Watch the area just in front of the ear, were the TMJ is located (a helpful technique is for the therapist to position index fingers on the TMJ while patient opens and closes jaw). This technique will help you assess which side is deviating.
2 Palpate pterygoid muscles at the TMJ and have client open and close the mandible to feel for any deformities, popping, or grinding on a specific side.

POSITION: CLIENT IS NOW SUPINE

PROCEDURE:

1 Effleurage the masseter superior to inferior.
2 Perform thumb-stripping (with-fiber friction) on the same area from the TMJ toward the mandible (Figure 7-1).

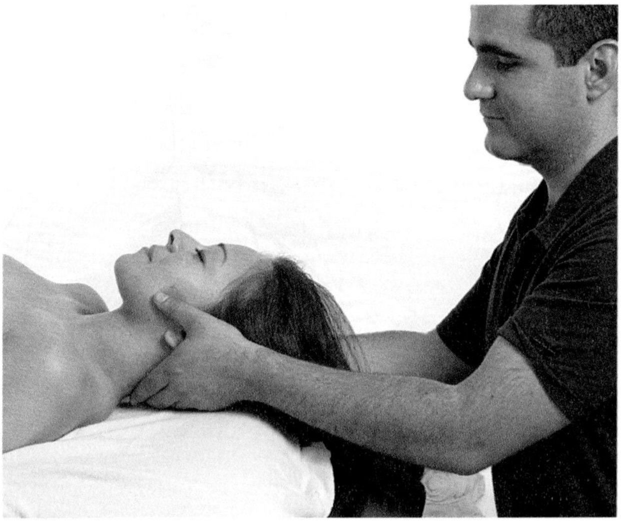

FIGURE 7-1

TEMPORAL MANDIBULAR JOINT ROUTINE

3 Perform cross-fiber friction on the area just below the TMJ (origin).

NOTE: Friction origin only!

4 Once the area is warmed up perform trigger point therapy on the origin of the masseter.

5 Gently perform hair-pulling to release temporalis muscle.

6 Put on latex gloves (dip index finger of glove in mouthwash to neutralize the taste of latex).

7 Pincer-grip the masseter with one finger inside the mouth and the other on the outer part and compress the muscle 2 to 3 times from insertion to origin.

8 Continue to release pterygoid muscles by placing index finger in the TMJ capsule (between the cheek and the molars) and hold to release, having the client breathe in and out for a faster release.

NOTE: Mouth should be open half an inch.

9 Once released (finger will sink into capsule) start to look for trigger points. If any are found, apply friction to each one for 5 seconds.

10 Remove finger slowly.

11 Perform concluding strokes (effleurage and nerve strokes) to the outer portion of the cheeks.

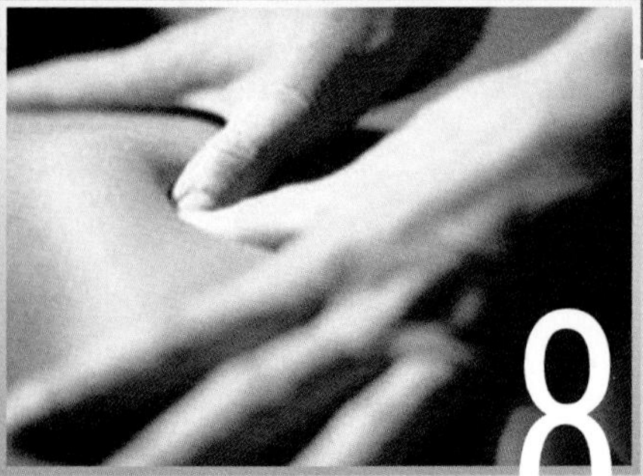

CHAPTER 8

THORACIC OUTLET SYNDROME (TOS)

OUTLINE

Definition and symptoms
Indications
Contraindications
Thoracic outlet syndrome routine

KEY TERM

Thoracic outlet syndrome

OBJECTIVES

Upon completion of this chapter the reader will have the information necessary to:

1. **Define common thoracic outlet syndrome causes**
2. **Describe common thoracic outlet syndrome symptoms**
3. **Identify common thoracic outlet syndrome routine indications**
4. **Classify common thoracic outlet syndrome routine contraindications**
5. **Understand and perform a thoracic outlet syndrome routine**

DEFINITION AND SYMPTOMS

Thoracic outlet syndrome (TOS) is a compression, injury, or irritation to the neurovascular structures located at the root of the neck or upper thoracic region (thoracic outlet). This disorder is often the result of entrapment of the neurovascular structures by the anterior and middle scalene muscles between the clavicle and first rib, possible hypotrophy or hypertrophy of the subclavius, or entrapment by the pectoralis minor muscle.

Common complaints include pain, numbness, tingling, and heaviness of the affected upper extremity leading to neck pain and headaches. Female clients are often diagnosed more commonly with TOS than males (female-to-male ratio is approximately 9 : 1). The shape of the chest wall in women is believed to influence this by encouraging closure of the thoracic outlet; large breasts

Icon represents an area where extreme caution should be used to avoid damage or compression to underlying or neighboring vessels.

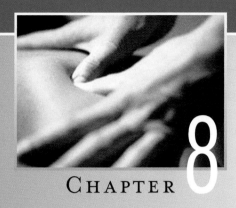

are often a cause, adding to the anterior forces on the chest, which leads to drooped shoulder posturing and further closing of the outlet. Pregnancy can also be a cause because of the postural adjustments the body goes through in a relatively short period of time.

Other known names for TOS are brachial plexopathy, cervicobrachial myofascial pain syndrome, cervicobrachial pain syndrome, costoclavicular mass syndrome, costoclavicular syndrome, scalenus anticus syndrome, scalenus syndrome, thoracic outlet compression syndrome, or cervical rib syndrome.

Indications

- Mechanical or postural disorders
- Stress
- Depression
- Overuse
- Kyphosis (see Chapter 16)
- For females: large chest
- Pregnancy (consult with physician before deciding on treatment)
- Subacute and chronic trauma
- Fibromyalgia (see Chapter 28)

Contraindications

- Vascular lesions
- Thrombus
- Aneurysms
- Fractures
- Edema
- Embolism
- Tumors
- Infections

THORACIC OUTLET SYNDROME ROUTINE

POSITION: CLIENT IS PRONE

PROCEDURE:

1 Effleurage and petrissage the entire posterior cervical, trapezius, rhomboids, and levator scapulae muscles.
2 Focus on affected side; perform with-fiber stripping on the upper and middle trapezius. This technique can be performed starting laterally to the spine and stripping outward toward the scapula.
3 Treat all active trigger points found on the upper trapezius, levator scapulae, and supraspinous muscles.
4 Perform upper trapezius stretch (L shape) by placing one hand on the occipital region and the other on the shoulder. Hold for 5 to 10 seconds (Figures 8-1 and 8-2).

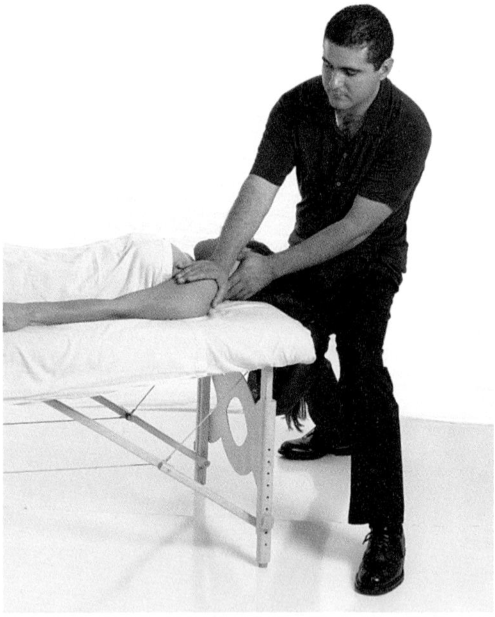

FIGURE 8-1 ■ Perform upper Trapezius stretch (L shape) by placing one hand on occipital region and the other on the shoulder.

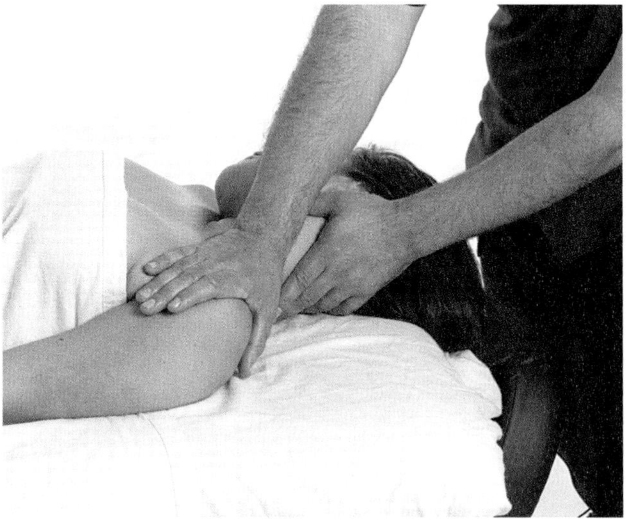

Figure 8-2 ■ Hold for 5-10 seconds.

POSITION: CLIENT IS NOW SUPINE

PROCEDURE:

1 Cradle head with both hands and with the tips of the fingers perform cross-fiber friction one side at a time on the occipital ridge (Figure 8-3).

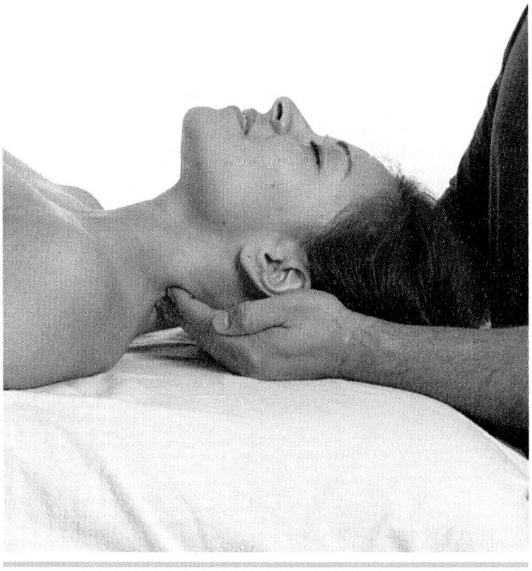

Figure 8-3 ■

THORACIC OUTLET SYNDROME ROUTINE

2 Release splenius capitis and cervices by performing thumb-stripping on the cervical area one side at a time along the lamina groove.

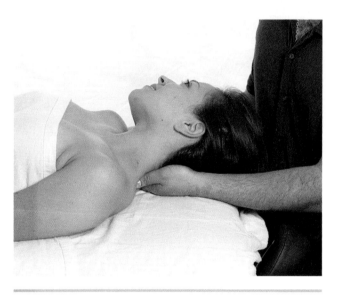

FIGURE 8-4

3 With caution, strip the scalene muscles (posterior to the sternocleidomastoid muscle), looking for active trigger points. If any are found, treat accordingly until they are deactivated (Figure 8-5).

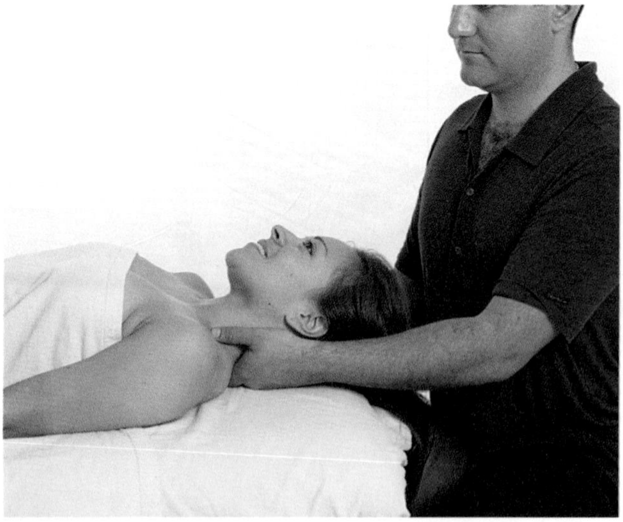

FIGURE 8-5

THORACIC OUTLET SYNDROME ROUTINE

4 Stretch cervical region by moving head to the side (ear to shoulder) followed by stretching head forward (chin toward chest). Perform stretches twice.
5 Effleurage under the clavicle and perform myofascial release (MFR, pumping) on pectoralis muscle (Figure 8-6).

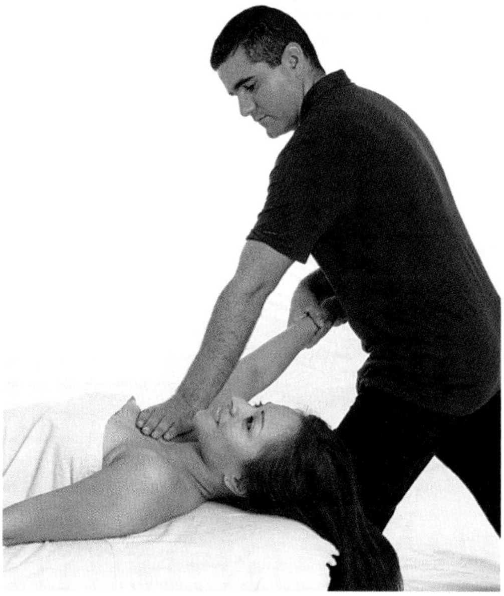

FIGURE 8-6 ■

6 Once the area is warmed up, perform with-fiber friction and trigger point therapy on the pectoralis minor.
7 Effleurage the entire area.
8 Perform pectoralis stretch after patient is dressed.

NOTE: If TOS is severe, displace the trachea, refer to the migraine treatment routine in Chapter 6, and release anterior scalene muscles.

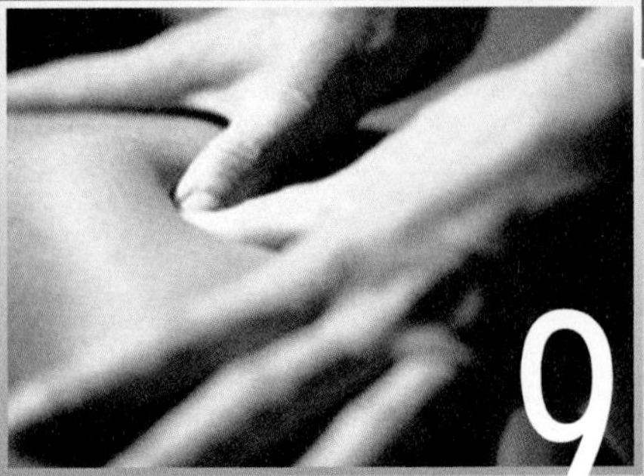

CHAPTER 9

TORTICOLLIS

OUTLINE

Definition and symptoms
Indications
Contraindications
Torticollis routine

KEY TERMS

Torticollis
Proprioceptive neuromuscular facilitation

OBJECTIVES

Upon completion of this chapter the reader will have the information necessary to:

1. **Define common torticollis causes**
2. **Describe common torticollis symptoms**
3. **Identify common torticollis routine indications**
4. **Classify common torticollis routine contraindications**
5. **Understand and perform a torticollis routine**

DEFINITION AND SYMPTOMS

Torticollis (wry neck)–a congenital or acquired condition of limited neck motion in which the person holds the head to one side with the chin pointing to the opposite side. It is the result of the shortening of the sternocleidomastoid (SCM) muscle. In early infancy (of the condition), a firm, nontender mass may be felt in the belly of the muscle and if left untreated, it can lead to permanent limitation of range of motion (ROM). Symptoms can last for as long as three weeks. Various treatments for wry neck are gentle stretching exercises, injections, pain killers, or massage therapy.

Icon represents an area where extreme caution should be used to avoid damage or compression to underlying or neighboring vessels.

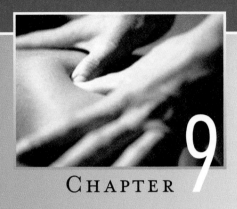

If the client agrees, **proprioceptive neuromuscular facilitation** (PNF) would be beneficial immediately following the treatment. PNF is method of stretching your body that involves the neuromuscular mechanism via the proprioceptors. Proprioceptors are responsible for the monitoring of tension and stretch, sending feedback to your brain. This style of stretching takes the muscle through a stretch (an 8 on a scale of 1-10 in pain), followed by an isometric contraction (hold for 8-10 seconds), which is immediately followed by a final stretch.

Indications

- Stiff neck
- Limited ROM
- Poor posture
- "Kink in the neck"
- Poor sleep history

Contraindications

- Acute herniated cervical discs
- Trauma
- Edema
- Skin rash
- History of stroke (consult a physician)

TORTICOLLIS ROUTINE

POSITION: CLIENT IS SUPINE

PROCEDURE:

1 Effleurage the shoulders and posterior neck muscles.
2 Petrissage the client's posterior neck muscles (lightly lubricated), concentrating on the upper trapezius (massage both sides).
3 Hold head with one hand and thumb-strip next to the lamina groove using the other hand.
4 Apply cross-fiber friction and with-fiber friction to the occipital ridge (Figure 9-1).

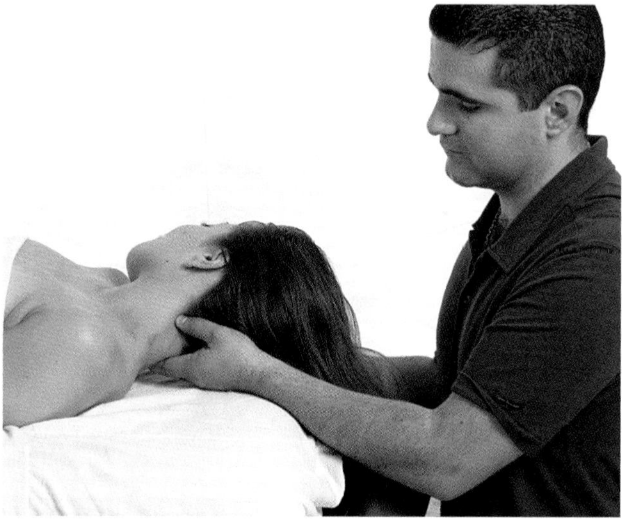

FIGURE 9-1 ■

5 Gently perform occipital release (manual head traction) and hold for 15 to 20 seconds.
6 With caution, strip the scalene muscles (posterior to the SCM) looking for active trigger points. If any are found, treat them accordingly until they are deactivated.
7 Pincer-grip the levator scapula and apply thumb-stripping (perform technique to both sides).

8 Skin-roll platysma muscle bilaterally (Figure 9-2).

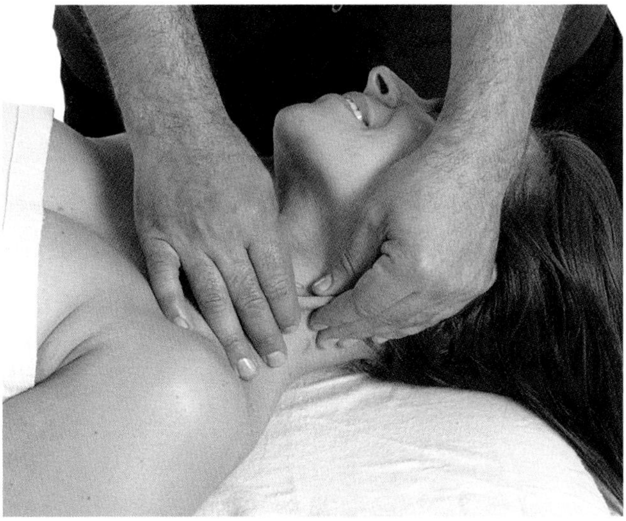

FIGURE 9-2

9 Locate the SCM and lightly lubricate (have client slightly lift head if muscle is difficult to find).
10 Thumb-strip the SCM from insertion to origin.
11 Apply pincer grip and with-fiber friction by performing the money sign (Figure 9-3).

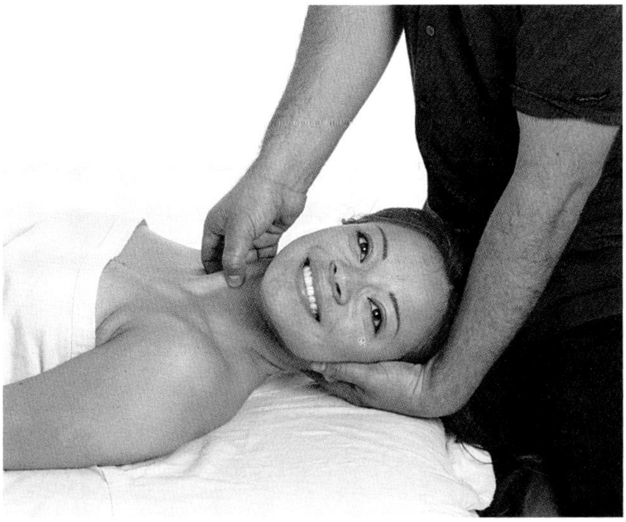

FIGURE 9-3

12 Use cross-fiber friction on the origin and insertion of the SCM (at clavicular head make sure to use friction under the clavicle only after client exhales).

13 Repeat steps 8 through 11 on the other SCM.

14 Find and deactivate all active trigger points on the trapezius (Figure 9-4).

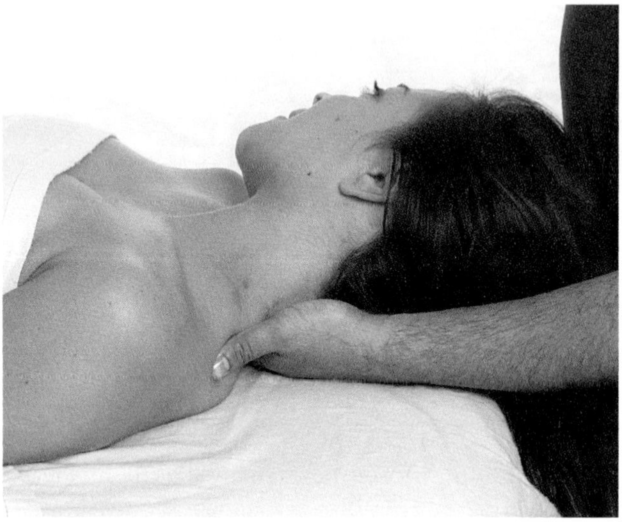

FIGURE 9-4

TORTICOLLIS ROUTINE

15 Pincer-grip the upper trapezius muscles to include serratus posterior superior (Figure 9-5).

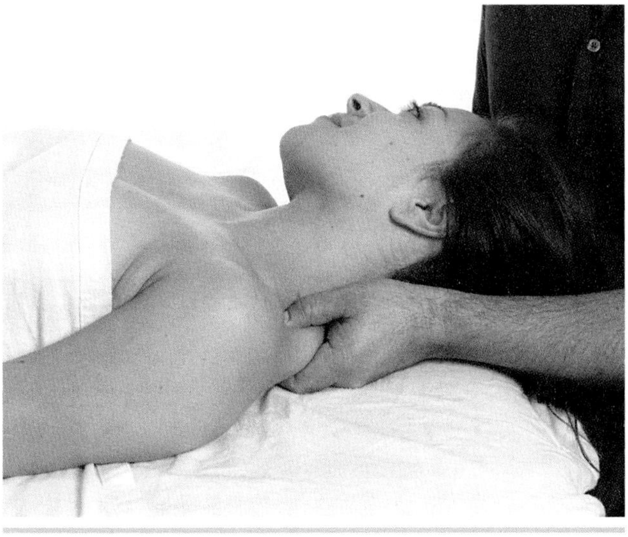

FIGURE 9-5

16 Effleurage the area and perform concluding strokes.
17 Complete the treatment by performing lateral and head-to-chest stretches.

NOTE: PNF technique may be used only if the client agrees.

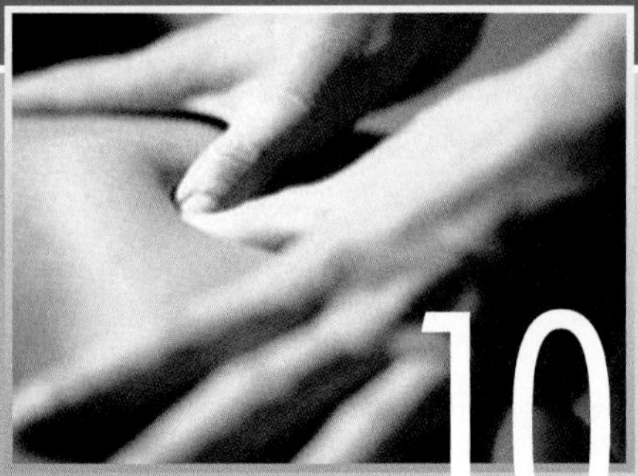

CHAPTER 10

WHIPLASH

OUTLINE

Definition and symptoms
Indications
Contraindications
Whiplash routine

KEY TERMS

Whiplash
Sub-acute whiplash
Chronic whiplash

OBJECTIVES

Upon completion of this chapter the reader will have the information necessary to:

1. **Define common whiplash causes**
2. **Describe common whiplash symptoms**
3. **Identify common whiplash routine indications**
4. **Classify common whiplash routine contraindications**
5. **Understand and perform a whiplash routine**

DEFINITION AND SYMPTOMS

Whiplash is a soft-tissue injury to the neck that can also be known as neck sprain or neck strain. It is characterized by a set of symptoms that occur after damage to the neck, usually because of sudden extension and flexion (e.g., a rear-end car accident). Injury can involve intervertebral joints, discs, ligaments, cervical muscles, and nerve roots. Neck pain may not be present at the time of the accident but can appear soon after.

Other symptoms may include neck stiffness, injuries to the muscles and ligaments, headache, dizziness, abnormal sensations such as burning or paresthesia (numbness), or shoulder and back pain. In severe cases, the affected individual might have memory loss,

⚠ Icon represents an area where extreme caution should be used to avoid damage or compression to underlying or neighboring vessels.

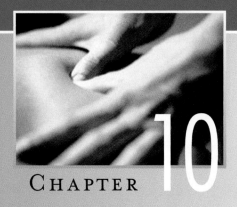

concentration impairment, nervousness/irritability, sleep disturbances, fatigue, or depression.

Indications

- **Sub-acute whiplash**
- **Chronic whiplash**
- Stiff neck
- Reduced range of motion

Contraindications

- Acute herniated discs
- Edema
- Skin conditions
- Dislocations
- Client taking heavy pain medication

WHIPLASH ROUTINE

POSITION: CLIENT IS SUPINE

PROCEDURE:

1 Effleurage the posterior cervical muscles by placing both hands under the neck and stroking upward toward the occipital ridge.
2 Perform petrissage to the posterior cervical muscles.
3 Perform cross-fiber friction on occipital ridge one side at a time (Figure 10-1).

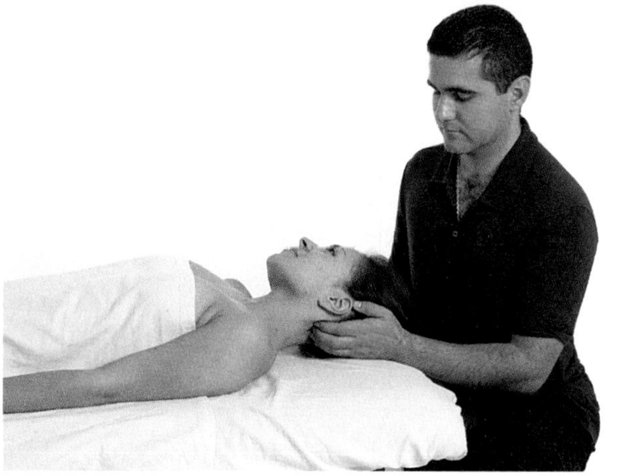

FIGURE 10-1

4 Perform trigger point therapy to the posterior cervical muscles.
5 Apply deep-stripping (scoop) on splenius capitis and cervices followed by stripping on the upper trapezius (Figure 10-2).

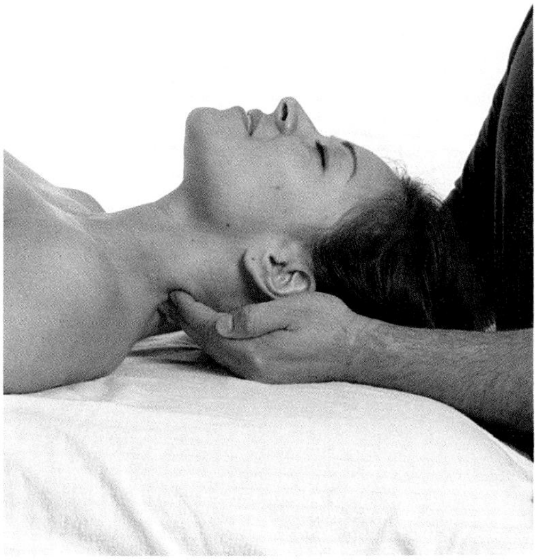

FIGURE 10-2 ■

6 Effleurage the anterior neck.
7 Thumb-strip the scalene muscles on the anterior lateral neck area (behind the sternocleidomastoid [SCM] muscle) and feel for active trigger points.
8 Stretch neck to the opposite side worked.
9 Lightly effleurage anterior neck, looking for and deactivating active trigger points on the origin of the SCM muscle.

WHIPLASH ROUTINE

10 Have the client look to the opposite side being worked and lift head. This will make it easier to pincer-grip the SCM muscle. Move from superior (mastoid process) to inferior (clavicle), making the money sign while holding the muscle between fingers (Figure 10-3).

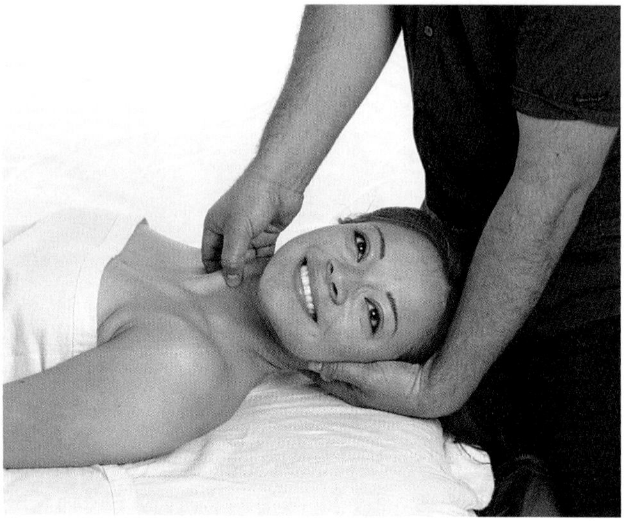

FIGURE 10-3 ■

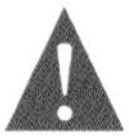

11 Find and deactivate all active trigger points on the SCM muscle (Figure 10-4).

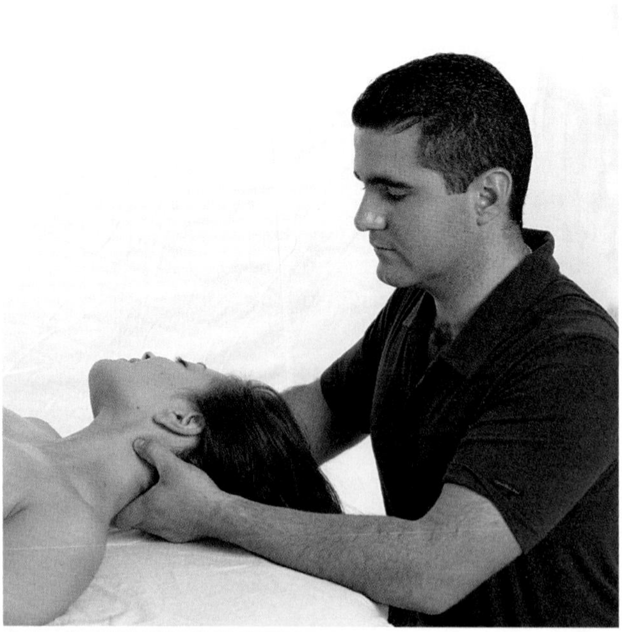

FIGURE 10-4 ■

12 Feather-stroke the anterior cervical muscles (Figure 10-5).

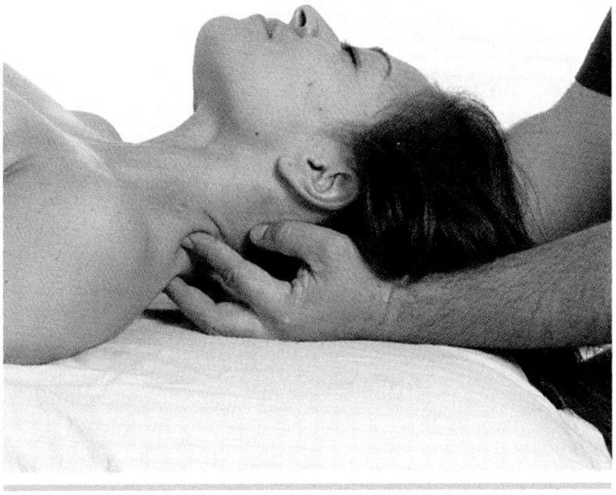

FIGURE 10-5

13 If scalene muscles have not released, displace the trachea to work on the anterior cervical muscles. Please refer to the migraine treatment routine in Chapter 6.

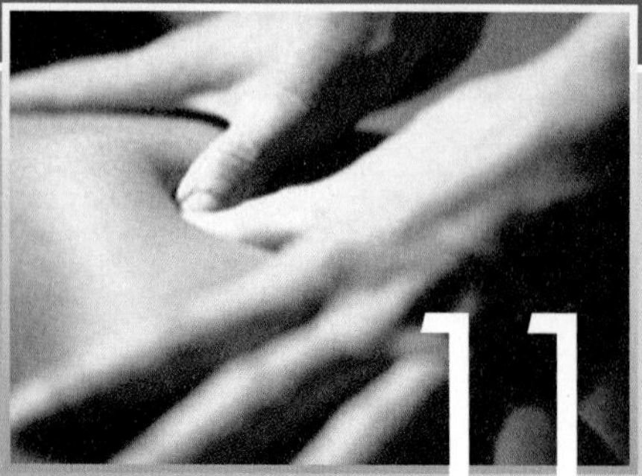

CHAPTER 11

FROZEN SHOULDER

OUTLINE

Definition and symptoms
Indications
Contraindications
Frozen shoulder routine

KEY TERMS

Frozen shoulder

OBJECTIVES

Upon completion of this chapter the reader will have the information necessary to:

1. **Define common frozen shoulder causes**
2. **Describe common frozen shoulder symptoms**
3. **Identify common frozen shoulder routine indications**
4. **Classify common frozen shoulder routine contraindications**
5. **Understand and perform a frozen shoulder routine**

DEFINITION AND SYMPTOMS

Frozen shoulder is a tear or strain in the rotator cuff muscles and/or tendons resulting in reduced range of motion (ROM). Degeneration and general wear-and-tear are usually the two major causes for injury. Because tendons of the rotator cuff muscles receive very little oxygen and nutrients from blood supply, they are especially vulnerable to degeneration with aging; hence, it is common for the elderly to have shoulder problems. This lack of blood supply is also the reason why a shoulder injury can take a long time to heal. There are two common symptoms of a shoulder injury: pain and weakness. Pain is not always felt when a shoulder injury occurs, but most people who do feel pain report that it is a very vague pain that can be hard to pinpoint. The

Icon represents an area where extreme caution should be used to avoid damage or compression to underlying or neighboring vessels.

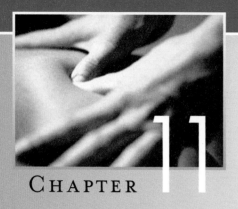

earlier a shoulder injury is treated the better. The first 48 to 72 hours, the subacute stage, are crucial to a complete and speedy recovery.

Indications

- Pain in the shoulder area
- Reduced range of motion (ROM)
- Scar tissue build-up
- Shoulder injuries
- Radiating pain

Contraindications

- Edema
- Peripheral vascular disease
- History of cancer
- Acute fractures

POSITION: CLIENT IS SUPINE

PROCEDURE:

1 Effleurage the pectoralis major.

2 Perform myofascial release (MFR, pumping technique) and compression on the pectoralis major (Figure 11-1).

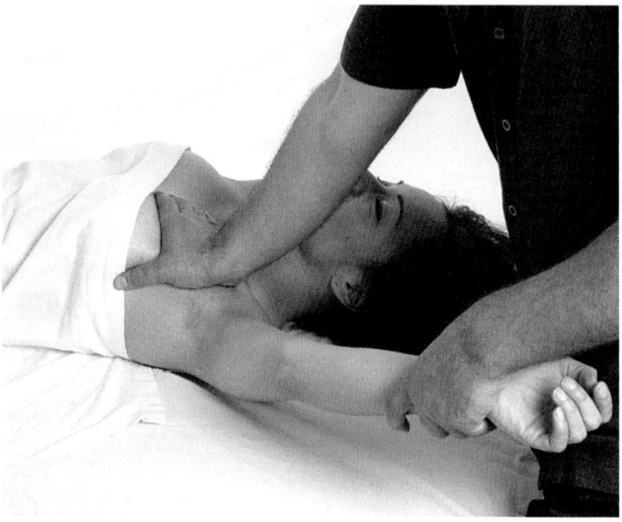

FIGURE 11-1 ■

3 Pincer-grip the pectoralis major from medial to lateral (Figures 11-2 and 11-3).

FROZEN SHOULDER ROUTINE

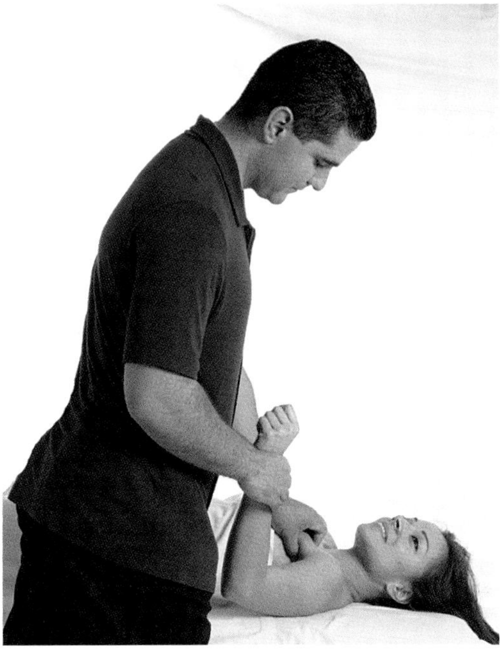

FIGURE 11-2 ■ Pincer grip pectoralis major, starting medial.

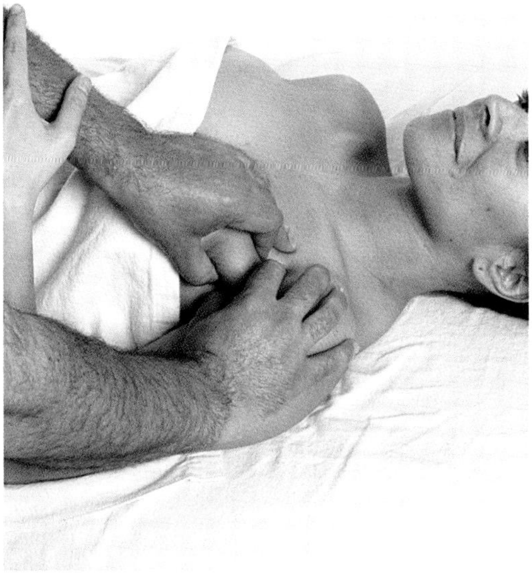

FIGURE 11-3 ■ Pincer grip pectoralis major, ending lateral.

FROZEN SHOULDER ROUTINE

4 Find any active trigger points on the pectoralis major and deactivate them.
5 Thumb-strip the pectoralis minor from superior to inferior (Figure 11-4).

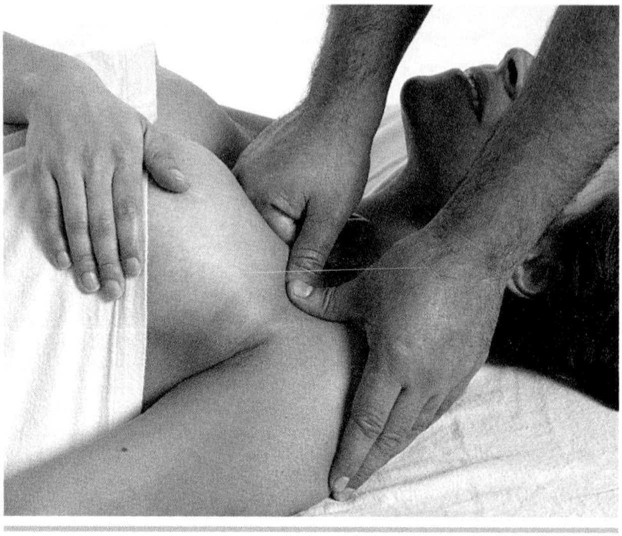

FIGURE 11-4 ■

6 Place palm over the shoulder joint and stroke toward the elbow. Use MFR on the deltoids, being careful not to exert too much pressure on the acromioclavicular joint.

POSITION: CLIENT IS NOW PRONE

PROCEDURE:

1 Effleurage the tissues and entire back.
2 Thumb-spread (with-fiber friction) the supraspinatus, levator scapula, and infraspinatus muscles.
3 Search for and deactivate all active trigger points on the levator scapula, supra, and infraspinatus muscles of the affected shoulder.

⚠ *Use caution with the radial nerve that runs in the area under the spine of the scapula.*

POSITION: CLIENT MOVES TO SIDE-LYING POSITION

PROCEDURE:

1 Effleurage the entire axillary area.
2 Place client's arm in abduction and thumb-spread (with-fiber friction) the teres minor (Figure 11-5).

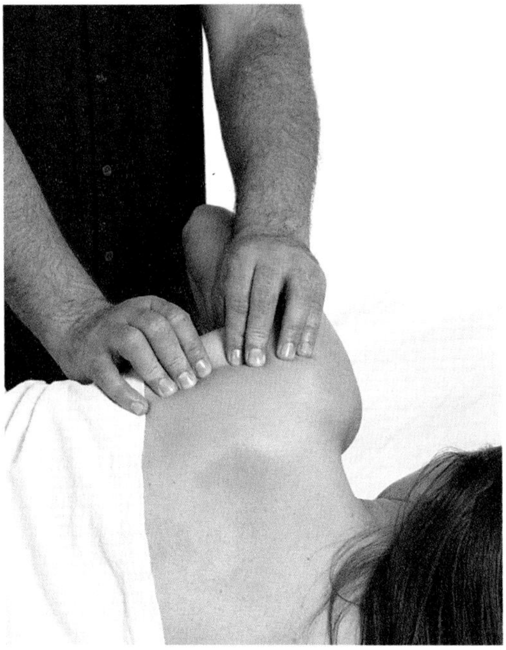

FIGURE 11-5 ■

3 If any active trigger points are encountered on the teres muscles, carefully deactivate them.
4 While client is still supporting arm, thumb-spread and use MFR (with palm) on the serratus anterior muscle area along the axillary border (Figure 11-6).

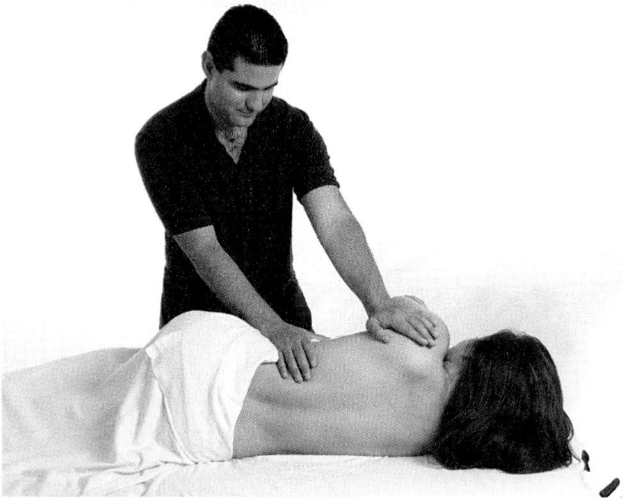

FIGURE 11-6 ■

FROZEN SHOULDER ROUTINE

5 Pull the shoulder forward at an angle and apply friction (with thumb) on the subscapularis muscle under the axillary border, being careful not to exceed patient's pain tolerance (not more than 8 on a 1-10 scale) (Figures 11-7 and 11-8).

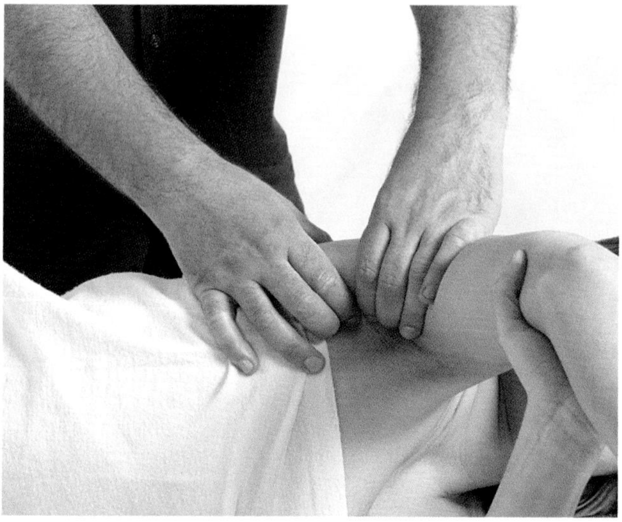

FIGURE 11-7 ■ Pull shoulder forward at an angle and apply friction with thumb on the subscapularis muscle under the axillary border: close-up view.

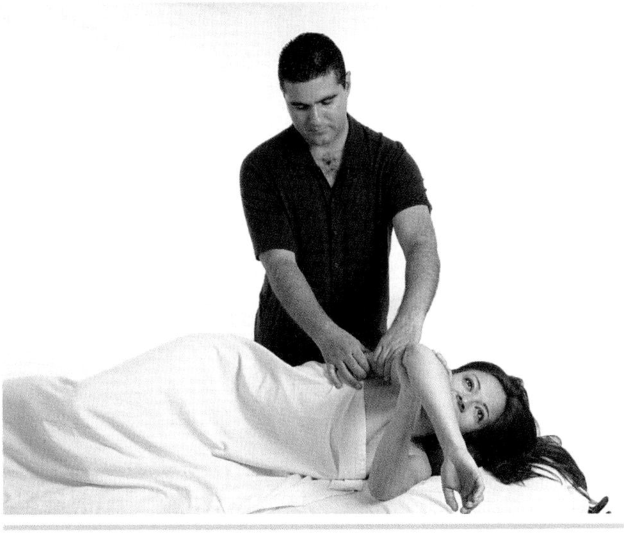

FIGURE 11-8 ■ Pull shoulder forward at an angle and apply friction with thumb on the subscapularis muscle under the axillary border: wide view.

6 Effleurage the entire area.
7 Conclude by performing rotator cuff stretches.

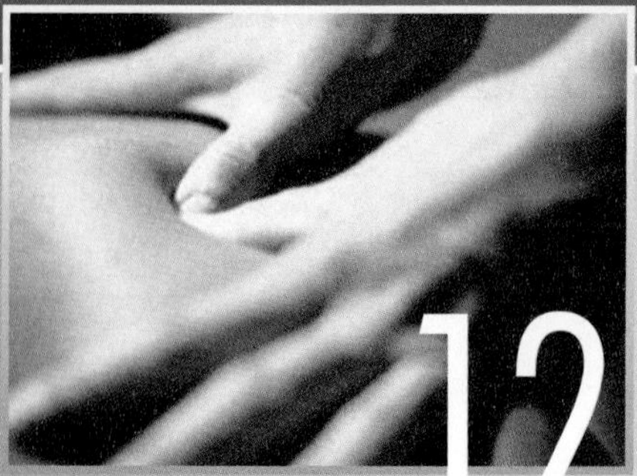

CHAPTER 12

ROTATOR CUFF

OUTLINE

Definition and symptoms
Indications
Contraindications
Rotator cuff routine

KEY TERMS

Rotator cuff tear

OBJECTIVES

Upon completion of this chapter the reader will have the information necessary to:

1. **Define common rotator cuff tear causes**
2. **Describe common rotator cuff tear symptoms**
3. **Identify common rotator cuff tear routine indications**
4. **Classify common rotator cuff tear routine contraindications**
5. **Understand and perform a rotator cuff tear routine**

DEFINITION AND SYMPTOMS

A **rotator cuff tear** is a tear in one of the four rotator cuff muscles or their tendons. The four muscles–supraspinatus, infraspinatus, teres minor, and subscapularis (SITS)–originate from the scapula and together form a single tendon unit that form a "cuff" over the upper end of the arm (head of the humerus). The rotator cuff helps lift and rotate the arm and stabilize the ball of the humerus within the joint. Symptoms of a rotator cuff tear may develop acutely or have a more gradual onset. Acute trauma is usually brought on by a lifting injury or a fall on the affected arm; however, onset is gradual and may be caused by repetitive activity or by degeneration of the tendon. A client with a rotator cuff tear might feel pain in the front of the shoulder that radiates down the side of the arm. Other symptoms may include stiffness, loss of motion, and loss of range of motion (ROM).

Treatment options may include:

- Deep tissue massage
- Rest and limited overhead activity
- Use of a sling to limit motion
- Anti-inflammatory medication
- Steroid injection
- Strengthening exercise and physical therapy

Indications

- Stiff shoulder
- Limited ROM
- Radiating pain
- Difficulty abducting arm
- Weakness

Contraindications

- Peripheral vascular disease (PVD)
- Third-degree tears
- Edema
- Throbbing sensation
- History of heart disease

POSITION: CLIENT IS SITTING IN A CHAIR

PROCEDURE:

1 Apply muscle testing to the affected arm by having client activate each rotator cuff individually (e.g., medial rotation, lateral rotation, abduction).

POSITION: CLIENT IS NOW SUPINE

PROCEDURE:

1 Warm up all shoulder muscles by performing effleurage.
2 Perform compression effleurage over the pectoralis major muscle, then pincer-grip 1-inch sections of the muscle from origin to insertion (Figures 12-1 and 12-2).

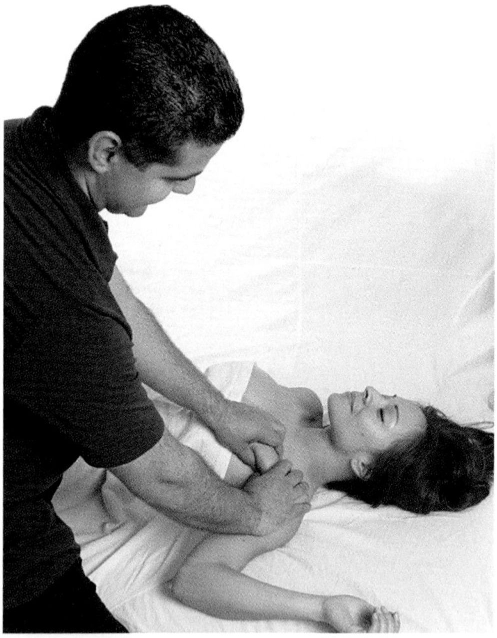

FIGURE 12-1 ■ Pincer gripping 1-inch sections of the pectoralis major muscle from origin to insertion: wide view.

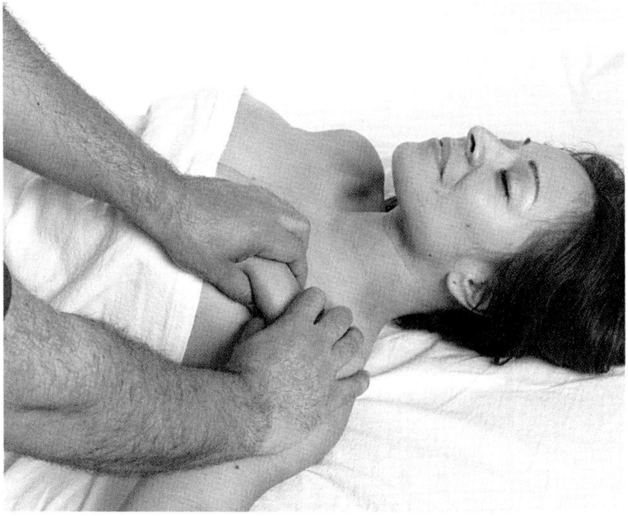

FIGURE 12-2 ■ Pincer gripping 1-inch sections of the pectoralis major muscle from origin to insertion: close-up view.

3 Perform transverse friction on the pectoralis major and subscapularis insertion (bicipital groove).
4 Execute the pectoralis major compression (pumping) 4 to 6 times until the area is hyperemic (Figure 12-3).

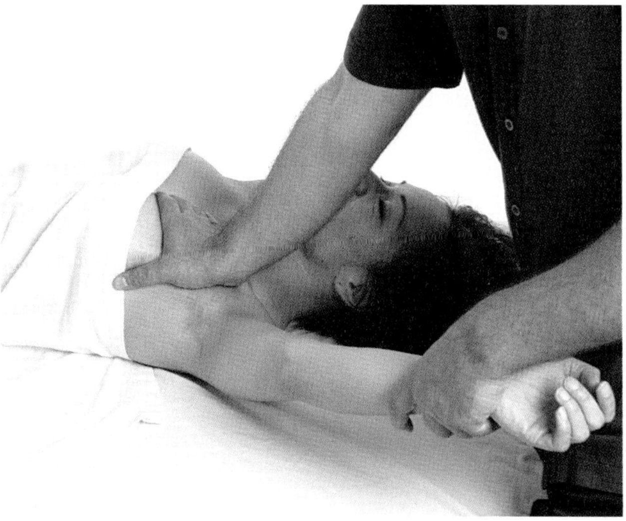

FIGURE 12-3 ■

POSITION: CLIENT IS NOW PRONE

1 Thumb-strip over the supraspinatus muscle from medial to lateral.
2 Perform friction (with-fiber and cross-fiber) on deep sections of the supraspinatus and infraspinatus muscles just posterior and medial to the acromioclavicular (AC) joint (Figures 12-4 and 12-5).

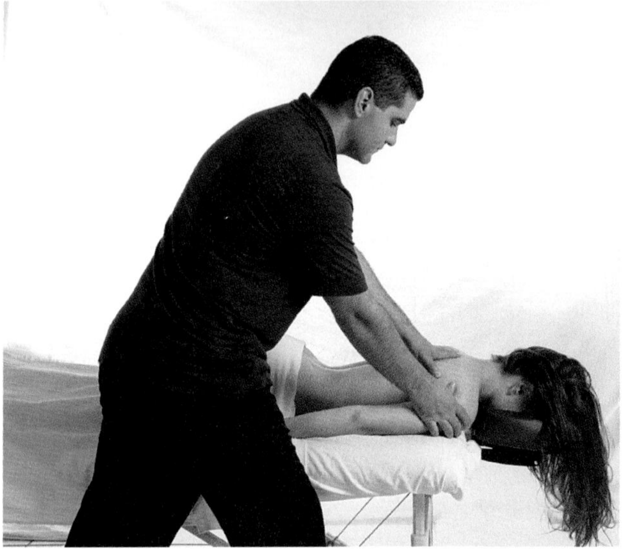

FIGURE 12-4 ■ This figure shows proper body mechanics while performing friction (with-fiber and cross-fiber) on deep sections of the supraspinatus and infraspinatus muscles just posterior and medial to the AC joint.

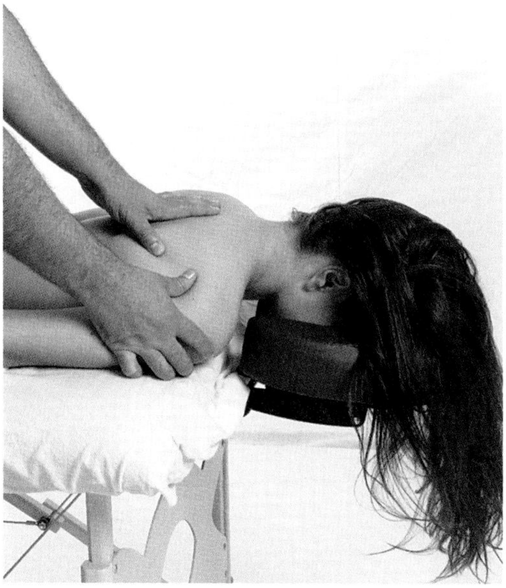

FIGURE 12-5 ■ A close-up of friction (with-fiber and cross-fiber) on deep sections of the supraspinatus and infraspinatus muscles just posterior and medial to the AC joint.

ROTATOR CUFF ROUTINE

3 Perform deep effleurage over infraspinatus, teres major, teres minor, and latissimus dorsi.
4 Use with-fiber friction on infraspinatus and teres minor.
5 Feel for active trigger points and deactivate them accordingly.
6 Perform cross-fiber friction on the SITS muscle tendons (Figure 12-6).

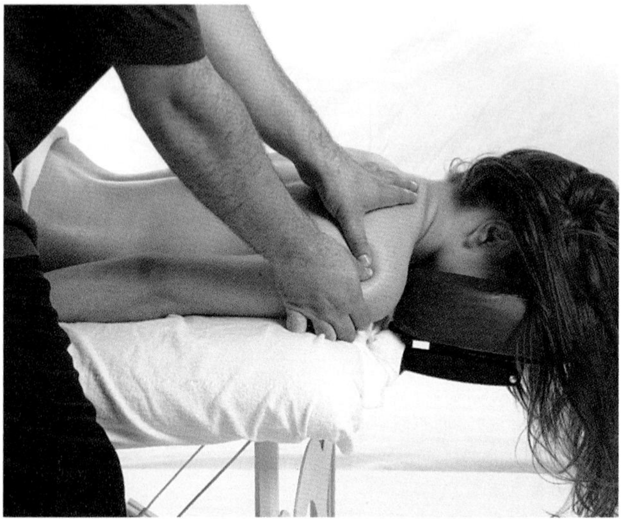

FIGURE 12-6

POSITION: CLIENT IS SIDE-LYING

PROCEDURE:

NOTE: Work on these muscles only if they were involved in the injury.

1 Effleurage the side from the lower ribs to just below the axilla.
2 Compress the teres major and latissimus dorsi and pincer-grip 1-inch sections.
3 Use with-fiber friction on the pectoralis minor from origin to insertion.
4 Have client prop up arm with the opposite arm. Stand in front of the client, pull shoulder forward, and apply thumb friction on the subscapularis muscle under the axillary border. Make sure to work within the client's pain threshold (not to exceed 8 on a 1-10 scale) (Figure 12-7).

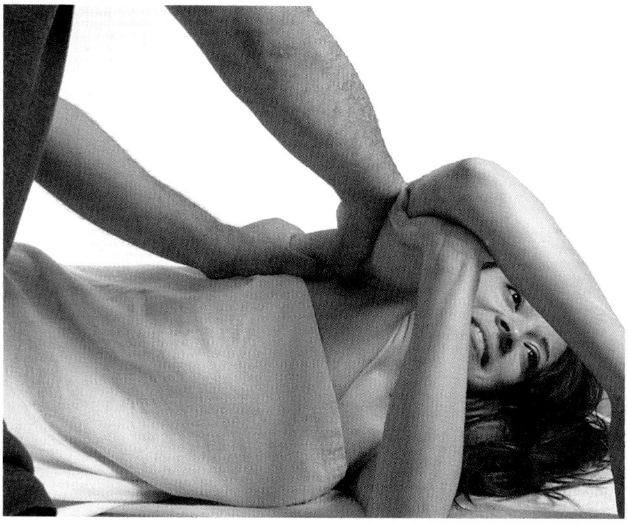

FIGURE 12-7

5 Perform ROM testing on the shoulder joint.
6 Pincer-grip the levator scapula and thumb-strip.
7 Conclude the treatment with effleurage and stretching of all rotator cuff muscles.

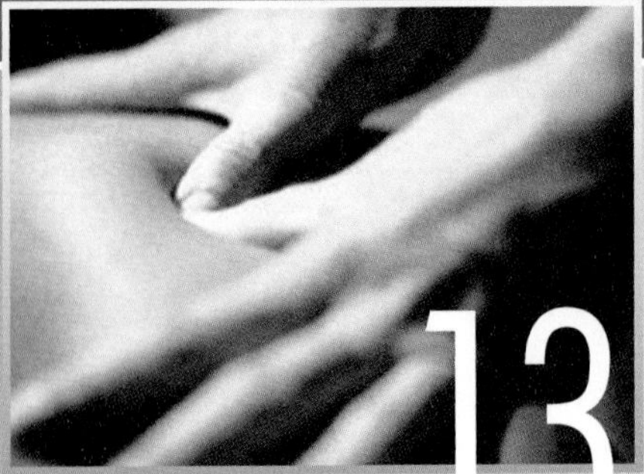

CHAPTER 13

LATERAL EPICONDYLITIS (TENNIS ELBOW)

OUTLINE

Definition and symptoms
Indications
Contraindications
Lateral epicondylitis routine

KEY TERMS

Lateral epicondylitis (tennis elbow)
Cryotherapy
T-bar

OBJECTIVES

Upon completion of this chapter the reader will have the information necessary to:

1. **Define common lateral epicondylitis (tennis elbow) causes**
2. **Describe common lateral epicondylitis (tennis elbow) symptoms**
3. **Identify common lateral epicondylitis (tennis elbow) routine indications**
4. **Classify common lateral epicondylitis (tennis elbow) routine contraindications**
5. **Understand and perform a lateral epicondylitis (tennis elbow) routine**

DEFINITION AND SYMPTOMS

Lateral epicondylitis (tennis elbow) is an inflammation or degeneration of the tendon that attaches to the lateral epicondyle of the humerus, an injury that is common among tennis players as a result of poor backhand technique or a too-small grip. A too-small grip means the muscles in the elbow must work harder, and they eventually become inflamed. The majority of people who get tennis elbow are between 40 and 50 years old, but it can affect athletes or non-athletes of any age. The symptoms for this injury are very similar to the entrapment of the radial nerve. Common treatments include the use of ultrasound or laser, massage therapy, rehabilitation, anti-inflammatory medication, steroid injection, or surgery (for pain lasting more than one year).

Some characteristics of lateral epicondylitis include:

- Pain in the outside of the elbow when the hand is bent back (extended) at the wrist, especially against resistance
- Pain on the outside of the elbow when trying to straighten the fingers against resistance
- Pain when lightly pressing on the lateral epicondyle of the humerus
- Weakness in the wrist

Indications

- Diagnosed lateral epicondylitis
- Reduced range of motion (ROM)
- "Annoying" pain in the elbow
- Pain radiating down the forearm
- Muscle weakness

Contraindications

- Severe edema
- Open lesions
- Peripheral vascular disorder (PVD)
- History of strokes
- History of heart disease (especially with left affected arm)

LATERAL EPICONDYLITIS (TENNIS ELBOW) ROUTINE

POSITION: CLIENT IS SUPINE OR SITTING WITH ARM OVER MASSAGE TABLE

PROCEDURE:

NOTE: ***Cryotherapy*** *(ice massage) may be used to numb the area.*

1 Place the client's hand in palm-dawn position and effleurage entire forearm.
2 Perform deep-stripping with palm on entire forearm. Stroke can be followed by deep palm-spreading.
3 Perform skin-rolling from medial to lateral (Figure 13-1).

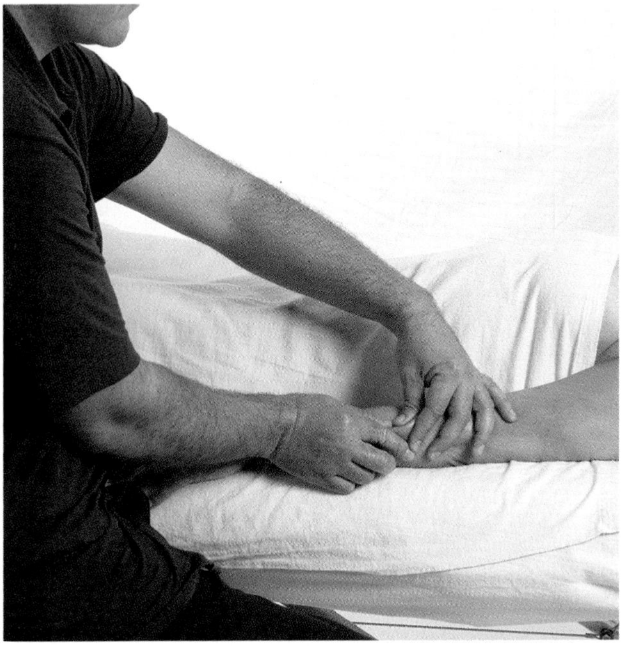

FIGURE 13-1

LATERAL EPICONDYLITIS (TENNIS ELBOW) ROUTINE

4 Perform deep thumb-stripping (with-fiber friction) from insertion to origin on extensors of the hand group. Make sure that all extensors of the hand (anterior and posterior) are worked (Figure 13-2).

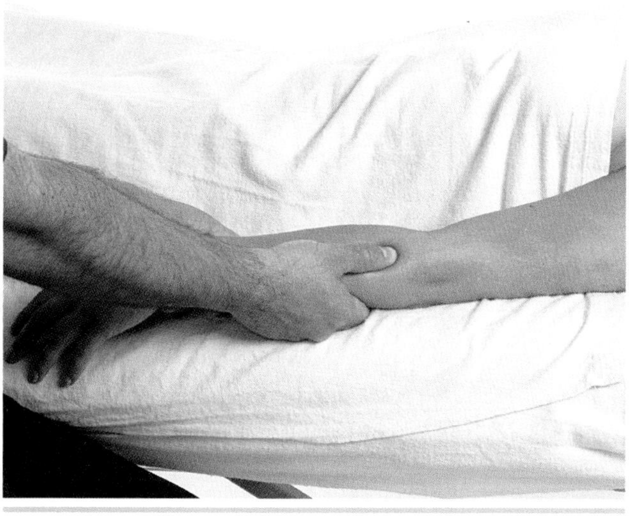

FIGURE 13-2

LATERAL EPICONDYLITIS (TENNIS ELBOW) ROUTINE

5 Release all active trigger points on the extensors of the hand group (especially the ones close to the lateral epicondyle).

6 Apply circular friction around the origin (lateral epicondyle of the humerus), being careful not to compress the nerves. The technique should be performed with an ice cube if area is inflamed (Figure 13-3).

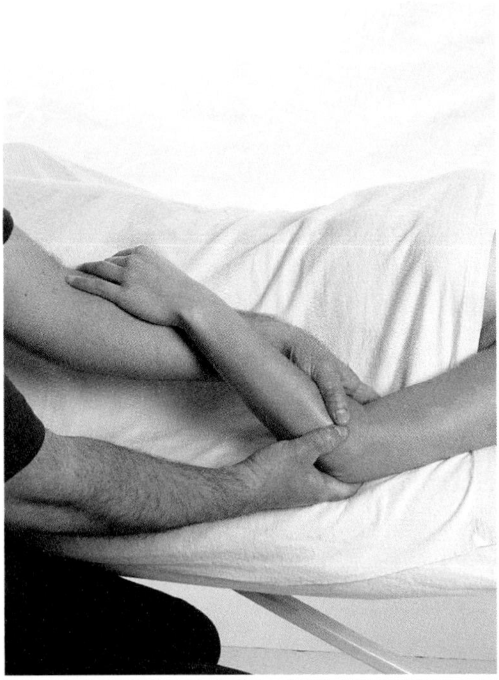

FIGURE 13-3

LATERAL EPICONDYLITIS (TENNIS ELBOW) ROUTINE

7 Perform one-hand petrissage on the biceps.
8 While flexing and extending the client's elbows, compress the biceps with the palm and spread upward (Figure 13-4).

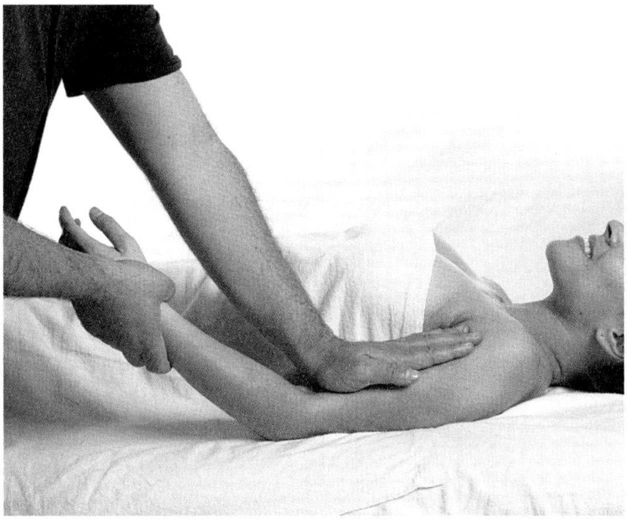

FIGURE 13-4

LATERAL EPICONDYLITIS (TENNIS ELBOW) ROUTINE

9 Perform one-hand petrissage on the triceps.
10 Hold the client's hand and medially rotate the forearm while placing thumb on the extensors (cross-fiber friction); continue technique to cover entire extensor group (Figure 13-5).

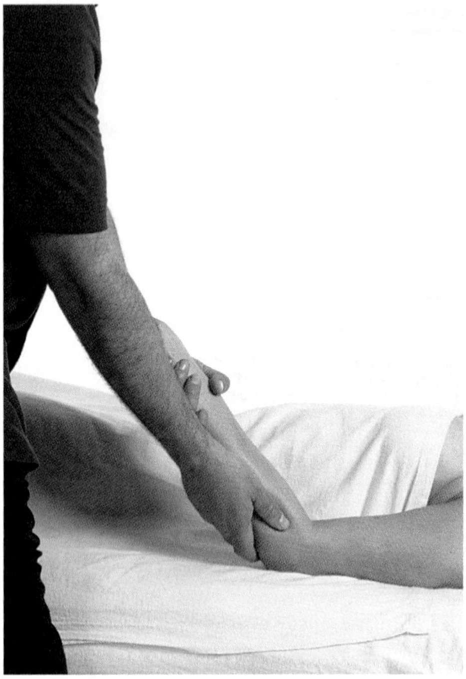

FIGURE 13-5

LATERAL EPICONDYLITIS (TENNIS ELBOW) ROUTINE

11 Perform thumb-gliding, stripping (with-fiber friction), and trigger point therapy on the client's palmar side of the hand (Figure 13-6).
*Note: A **T-bar** may be used.*

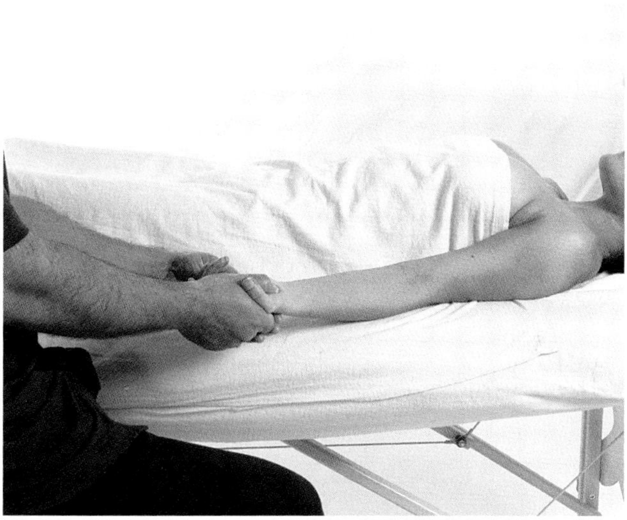

FIGURE 13-6

12 Include a good stretching and ROM session after treatment.

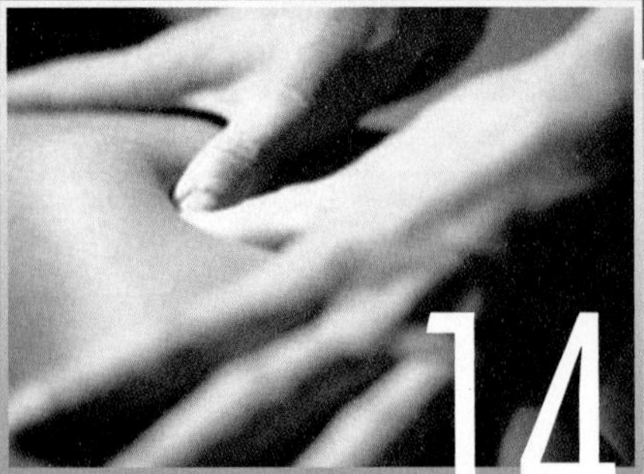

Chapter 14

MEDIAL EPICONDYLITIS (GOLFER'S ELBOW)

OUTLINE

Definition and symptoms
Indications
Contraindications
Medial epicondylitis (golfer's elbow) routine

KEY TERMS

Medial epicondylitis (golfer's elbow)

OBJECTIVES

Upon completion of this chapter the reader will have the information necessary to:

1. Define common medial epicondylitis (golfer's elbow) causes
2. Describe common medial epicondylitis (golfer's elbow) symptoms
3. Identify common medial epicondylitis (golfer's elbow) routine indications
4. Classify common medial epicondylitis (golfer's elbow) routine contraindications
5. Understand and perform a medial epicondylitis (golfer's elbow) routine

DEFINITION AND SYMPTOMS

Medial epicondylitis (golfer's elbow) is an inflammation or degeneration of the tendon that attaches to the medial epicondyle of the humerus. This injury can be caused by a forceful and repeated bending (flexing) of the wrist and fingers, causing tiny ruptures of the muscle and tendon in this area. Common causes for this injury include golfing, repeated bending (flexing) of the wrist, gripping, grasping, and turning the hand (overuse). Symptoms include tenderness and pain at the medial epicondyle, which is worsened by flexing the wrist. Common treatments include the use of anti-inflammatory medications, massage therapy, injections, and surgery. Often, resting the area at least 72 hours prevents further injury while allowing time to heal. Medial epicondylitis can be avoided by taking frequent breaks during work or play to improve overall arm muscle condition, stretching appropriately and limiting heavy pushing, pulling, or grasping.

Indications

- Diagnosed medial epicondylitis
- Reduced range of motion (ROM)
- "Annoying" pain in the elbow
- Pain radiating down the forearm
- Muscle weakness

Contraindications

- Severe edema
- Open lesions
- Peripheral vascular disorder (PVD)
- History of strokes
- History of heart disease (especially with left affected arm)

MEDIAL EPICONDYLITIS (GOLFER'S ELBOW) ROUTINE

POSITION: CLIENT IS SUPINE OR SITTING WITH ARM OVER MASSAGE TABLE

PROCEDURE:

NOTE: Cryotherapy (ice massage) may be used to numb the area.

1 Place the client's hand in supine position and effleurage entire forearm.
2 Perform deep-stripping with palm on entire forearm. Stroke can be followed by deep palm-spreading, focusing on the flexors of the hand (anterior forearm) group.
3 Perform skin-rolling from medial to lateral (Figure 14-1).

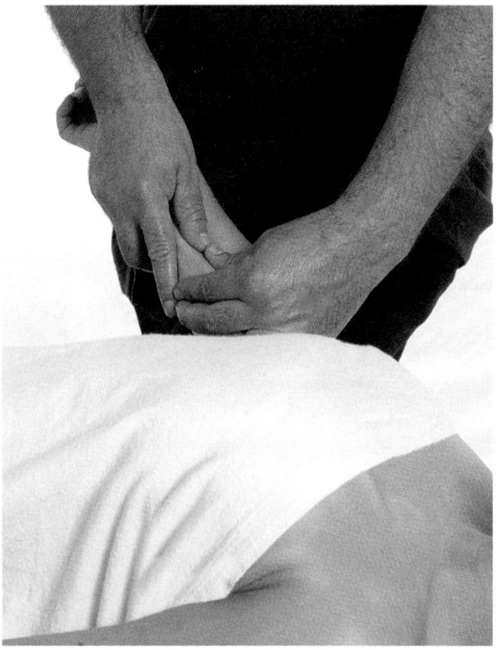

FIGURE 14-1

MEDIAL EPICONDYLITIS (GOLFER'S ELBOW) ROUTINE

4 Perform deep thumb-stripping (with-fiber friction) from insertion to origin on flexors of the hand group. Make sure that all flexors of the hand (anterior forearm) are worked (Figure 14-2).

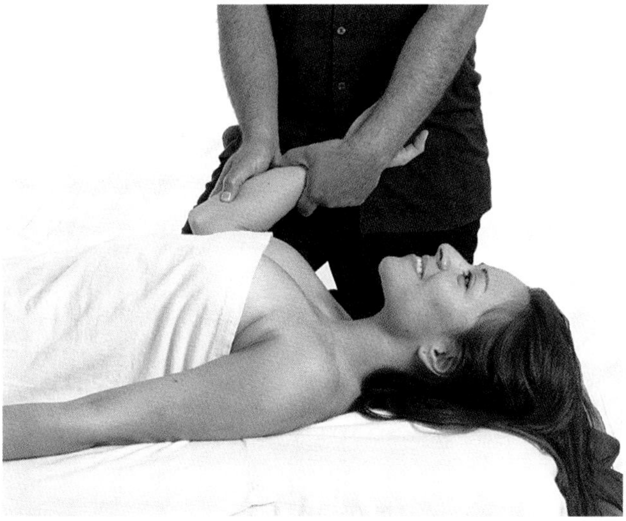

FIGURE 14-2

MEDIAL EPICONDYLITIS (GOLFER'S ELBOW) ROUTINE

5 Release all active trigger points on the flexors of the hand group (especially those close to the medial epicondyle).

⚠ 6 Apply circular friction around the origin (medial epicondyle of the humerus) with caution not to compress the nerves. The technique should be performed with an ice cube if the area is inflamed (Figure 14-3).

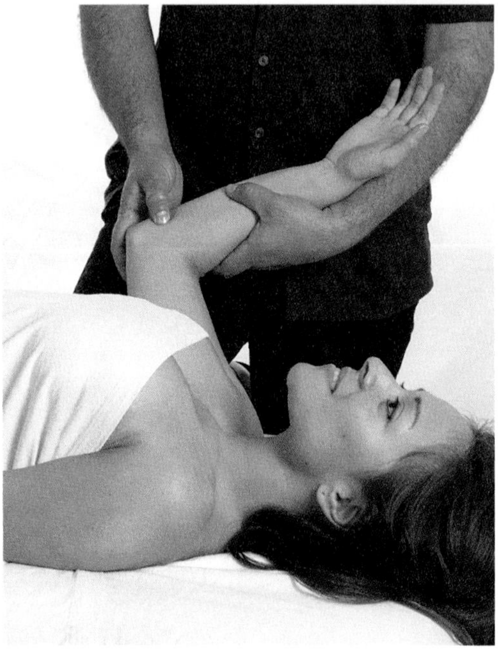

FIGURE 14-3

MEDIAL EPICONDYLITIS (GOLFER'S ELBOW) ROUTINE

7 Perform one-hand petrissage on the biceps.
8 While flexing and extending the client's elbows, compress the biceps with the palm and spread upward (Figure 14-4).

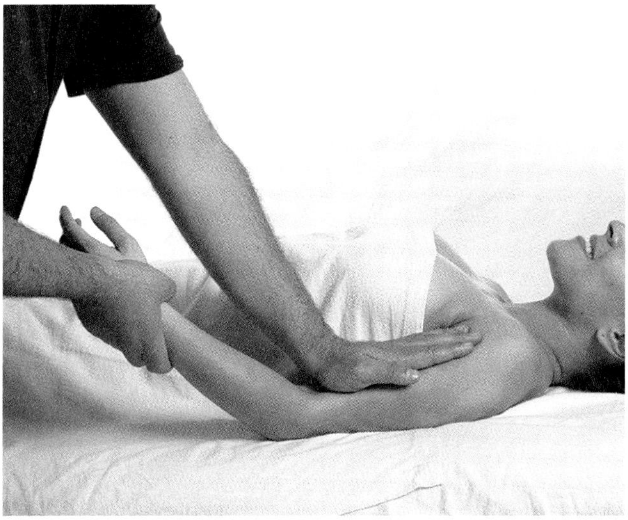

FIGURE 14-4

MEDIAL EPICONDYLITIS (GOLFER'S ELBOW) ROUTINE

9 Perform one-hand petrissage on the triceps.
10 Hold the client's hand and laterally rotate the forearm while placing thumb on the flexors (cross-fiber friction on the medial forearm); continue technique to cover entire flexor group (Figure 14-5).

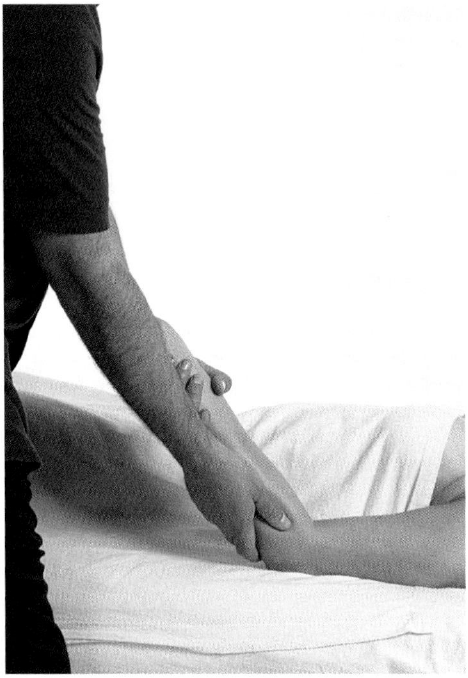

FIGURE 14-5

MEDIAL EPICONDYLITIS (GOLFER'S ELBOW) ROUTINE

11 Perform thumb-gliding, stripping (with-fiber friction), and trigger point therapy on the client's palmar side of the hand.

NOTE: A T-bar may be used.

12 Include a good stretching and ROM session after treatment.

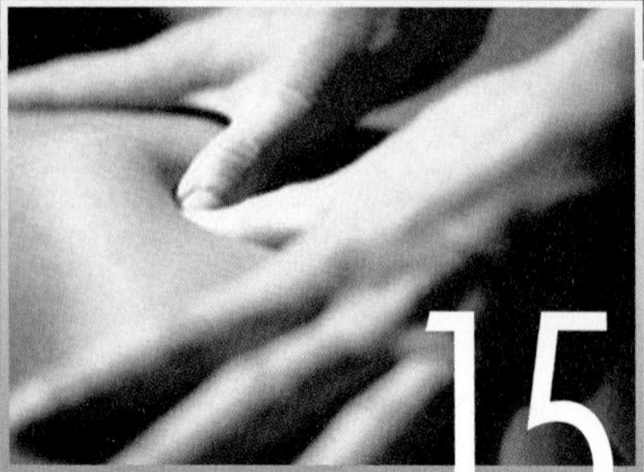

CHAPTER 15

CARPAL TUNNEL SYNDROME

OUTLINE

Definition and symptoms
Mechanics of carpal tunnel syndrome
Indications
Contraindications
Carpal tunnel syndrome routine

OBJECTIVES

Upon completion of this chapter the reader will have the information necessary to:

1. **Define common carpal tunnel syndrome (CTS) causes**
2. **Describe common CTS symptoms**
3. **Identify common CTS routine indications**
4. **Classify common CTS routine contraindications**
5. **Understand and perform a CTS routine**

KEY TERMS

Carpal tunnel syndrome
Ergonomics

DEFINITION AND SYMPTOMS

Carpal tunnel syndrome is a disorder in which the median nerve is compressed at the wrist causing symptoms such as burning, tingling, numbness in the fingers–especially the thumb, index, and middle fingers–and difficulty gripping or making a fist, which often causes dropping of things.

The median nerve runs through the carpal tunnel, a canal in the wrist surrounded by bone on three sides and a fibrous sheath (the flexor retinaculum) on the other. The median nerve, accompanied by many tendons leading toward the hand, runs through the carpal tunnel canal. The nerve can be compressed by swelling of the contents in the canal due to overuse (e.g., performing a repetitive task, such as typing) or other related neuromuscular disorders such as lateral and medial epicondylitis, TOS and frozen shoulder. Poor ergonomics, the study of designing objects in order to better adapt to the shape of the body or to correct a user's posture, can play a major role in the condition's onset.

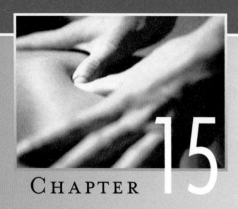

MECHANICS OF CARPAL TUNNEL SYNDROME

Carpal tunnel syndrome occurs when there is continuous pressure placed on the median nerve within the rigid, fixed space of the carpal tunnel, located between the carpal bones and the transverse carpal ligament of the wrist. The pressure reduces the volume of nerve impulses traveling to and from the hand. Mechanical pressure on the nerve can damage the nerve tissue (prolonged wrist flexion).

People often believe the only way to alleviate CTS is to have surgery, in which the flexor reticulum is cut to relieve the continuous pressure applied to the median nerve; however, the procedure is not always successful. Another solution is to inject steroids, such as cortisone, into the affected area. However, none of these invasive, extreme techniques is able to resolve the pressure problem like massage does.

The most common professions affected by this syndrome include massage therapists, information technology (IT) professionals, secretaries, factory workers, mechanics, and others who depend on repetitive hand movements. Carpal tunnel syndrome is often related to conditions such as tendonitis in the fingers ("trigger finger") or wrist. DeQuervain's tendonitis, for example, leads to pain in the wrist at the base of the thumb.

Indications

- Chronic pain
- Overuse
- Poor **ergonomics**
- Occupation-related
- Sports-related
- Repetitive strain injury

Contraindications

- Arthritis
- Fracture
- Osteoarthritis
- Visible skin conditions
- Lesions
- Edema
- Common massage contraindications

POSITION: CLIENT IS SUPINE

PROCEDURE:

NOTE: Cryotherapy (ice massage) may be used to numb the area.

1 Place the client's hand in supine position and effleurage the entire forearm.
2 Perform deep-stripping with palm on the entire forearm. The stroke can be followed by deep palm-spreading on entire forearm.
3 Perform skin-rolling from medial to lateral until the entire forearm has been skin-rolled (Figure 15-1).

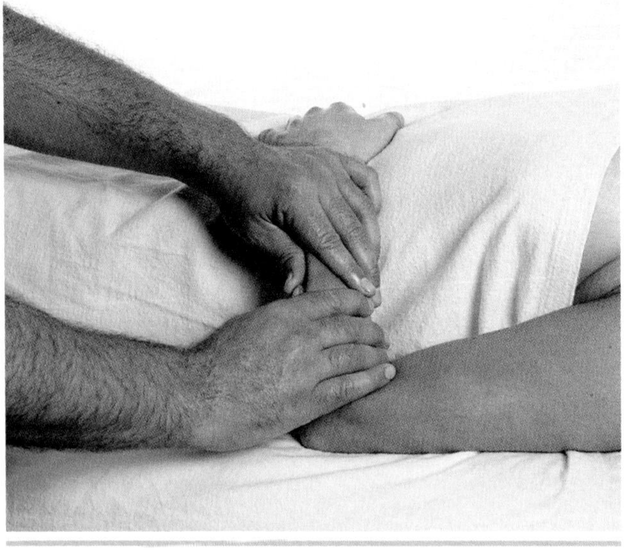

FIGURE 15-1 ■

4 Perform deep thumb-stripping (with-fiber friction) from insertion to origin on flexors and extensors of the hand groups.
5 Release all active trigger points on the extensors and flexors of the hand groups (especially the ones close to the medial and lateral epicondyle).
6 Apply circular friction around origin (medial and lateral epicondyle of the humerus) with caution not to compress nerves. The technique should be performed with an ice cube if the area is inflamed.

CARPAL TUNNEL SYNDROME ROUTINE

7 Thumb-strip (with-fiber friction) the tendons on the medial epicondyle of the humerus.

8 Flex client's arm at the elbow (90 degrees), therapist should place his/her arm on the client's bicep, interlock fingers with the client, and traction wrist. Technique may be assisted by using the other hand (therapist's hand) for extra traction force; however, be careful not to dislocate wrist (Figure 15-2).

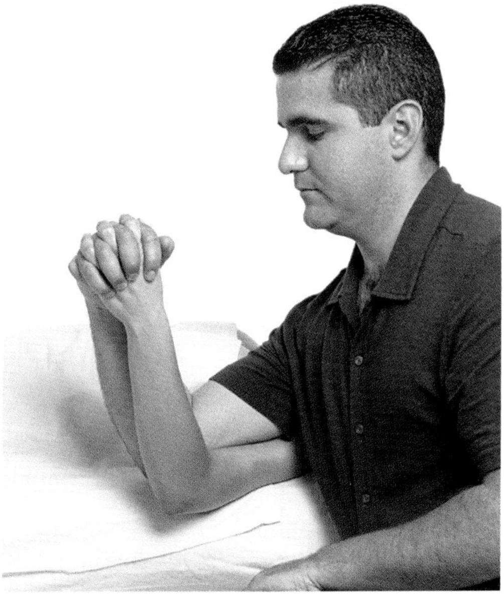

FIGURE 15-2

9 Use cross-fiber friction between each metacarpal. Use fingertips in small areas such as between the fourth and fifth metacarpal (Figure 15-3).

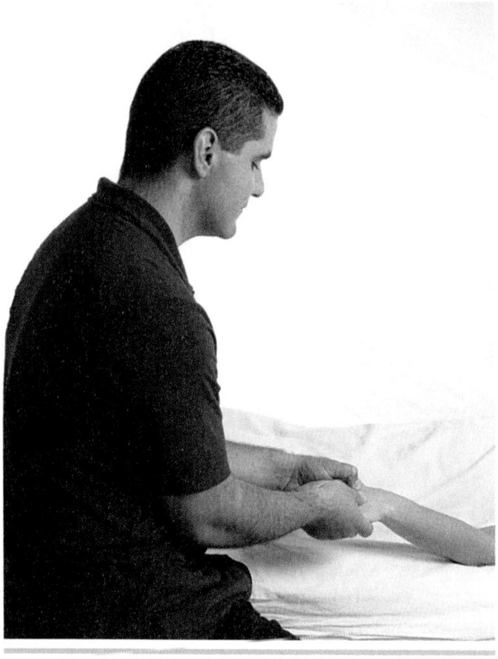

Figure 15-3 ■

10 Perform thumb-gliding, stripping (with-fiber friction) and trigger point therapy on the client's palmar side of the hand, making sure to reach in and around the pollicus muscles (Figure 15-4).

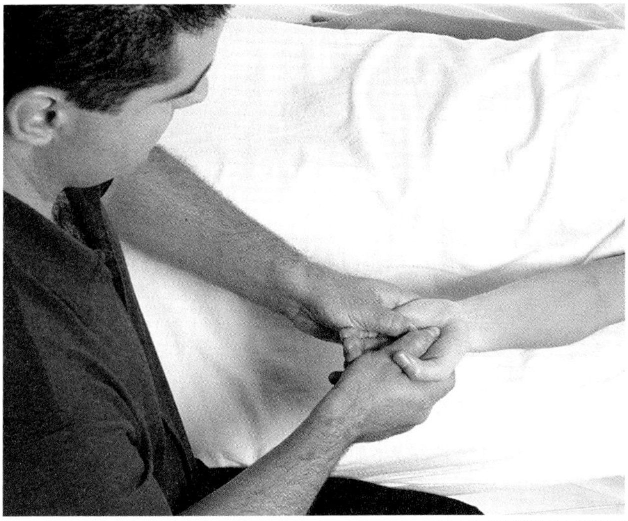

FIGURE 15-4

CARPAL TUNNEL SYNDROME ROUTINE

11 Perform one-hand petrissage on the biceps.
12 While flexing and extending the elbows, compress the biceps with the palm and spread upward.
13 Perform one-hand petrissage on the triceps.
14 Apply effleurage, myofascial release (MFR, pumping technique), and compression on the pectoralis major.
15 Pincer-grip the pectoralis major and uncoil using the money sign (Figure 15-5).

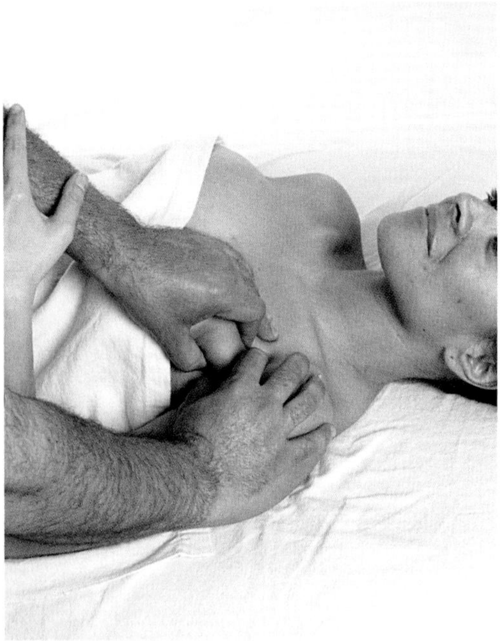

FIGURE 15-5 ■

CARPAL TUNNEL SYNDROME ROUTINE

16 Perform concluding strokes to the entire arm.
17 Make sure to include a good stretching and range of motion (ROM) session after treatment to all worked muscles.

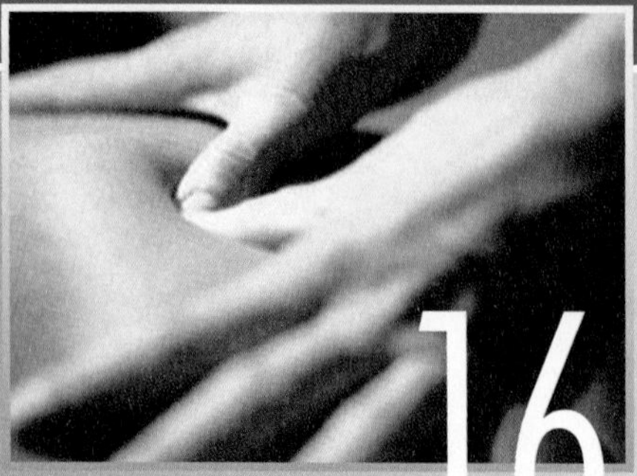

CHAPTER 16

KYPHOSIS

OUTLINE

Definition and symptoms
Indications
Contraindications
Kyphosis routine

KEY TERMS

Kyphosis
Postural kyphosis
Scheuermann's kyphosis
Congenital kyphosis

OBJECTIVES

Upon completion of this chapter the reader will have the information necessary to:

1 **Define common kyphosis causes**
2 **Describe common kyphosis symptoms**
3 **Identify common kyphosis routine indications**
4 **Classify common kyphosis routine contraindications**
5 **Understand and perform a kyphosis routine**

DEFINITION AND SYMPTOMS

Kyphosis is an exaggerated anterior concave curvature of the thoracic spine. The term *kyphosis* (ki-foe-sis) is usually applied to the curve that results in an exaggerated "round-back." Spinal x-rays allow physicians to measure the degree of the kyphotic curve. Any kyphotic curve that is more than 50 degrees is considered abnormal. The following are types of kyphosis:

Postural kyphosis. Most common, often attributed to "slouching." It is an exaggerated increase of the natural curve of the thoracic spine, which usually becomes noticeable during adolescence. More common among girls than boys.

Scheuermann's kyphosis. Named after the Danish radiologist who first described the condition, it presents significantly worse cosmetic deformity than postural kyphosis. Scheuermann's (shoe-er-mans) kyphosis usually affects the upper (thoracic) spine, but it can also occur in the lower (lumbar) spine. Aggravating factors include improper postural activity and long periods of standing or sitting.

Congenital kyphosis. Sometimes the spinal column does not develop properly while the fetus is in utero, resulting in the malformation of bones or the fusing together of several vertebrae. These abnormal situations may lead to progressive kyphosis as the infant grows, and surgical treatment may be needed at a very young age.

Indications

- Postural kyphosis
- Scheuermann's kyphosis
- For females: large chest (increasing anterior curvature)
- Poor posture
- Depression
- Rounded shoulders

Contraindications

- Aneurysms
- Heart conditions
- History of cancer

POSITION: CLIENT IS PRONE

PROCEDURE:

1 Effleurage and perform warm-up strokes on the entire back.
2 Palm-spread the erector spinae area from C7 down to T12 (Figure 16-1).

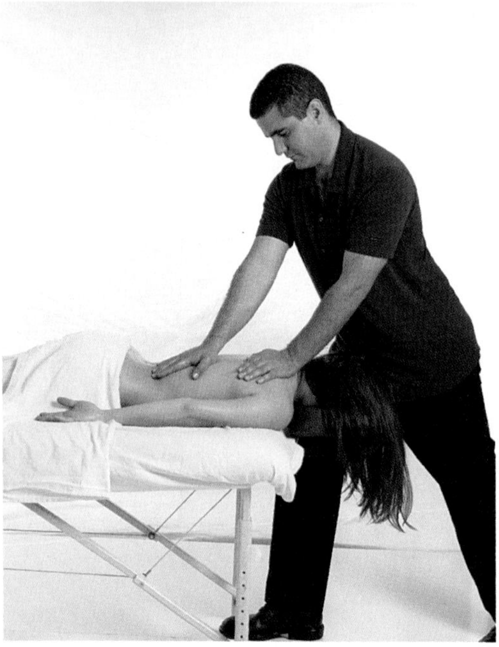

FIGURE 16-1

3 Skin-roll the back down to T12. Remember to work within the client's pain tolerance level (not to exceed 8 on a 1-10 scale).
4 Petrissage the posterior neck and shoulder muscles (upper trapezius, splenius cervicis and capitis, and levator scapulae).

5 Thumb-strip (with-fiber friction) from medial to lateral, beginning on the occipital ridge, and stripping down to the superior angle of the scapula.
6 Find and deactivate all active trigger points in the area. If knots are found, treat accordingly (Figure 16-2).

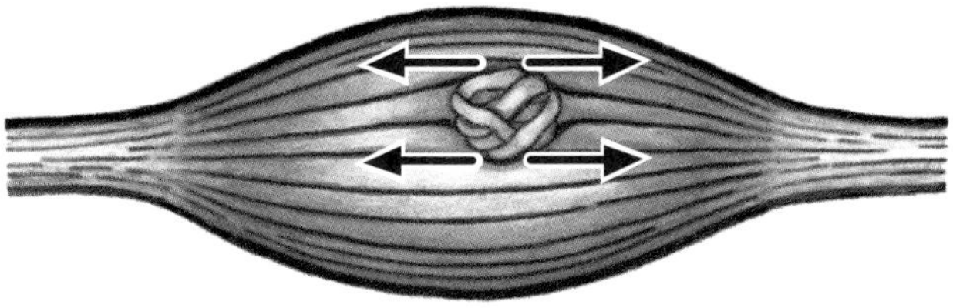

FIGURE 16-2 ■

7 Perform deep transverse and with-fiber friction on the origin (do not place too much pressure on the lamina groove) and insertion of the lower and middle trapezius (Figure 16-3).

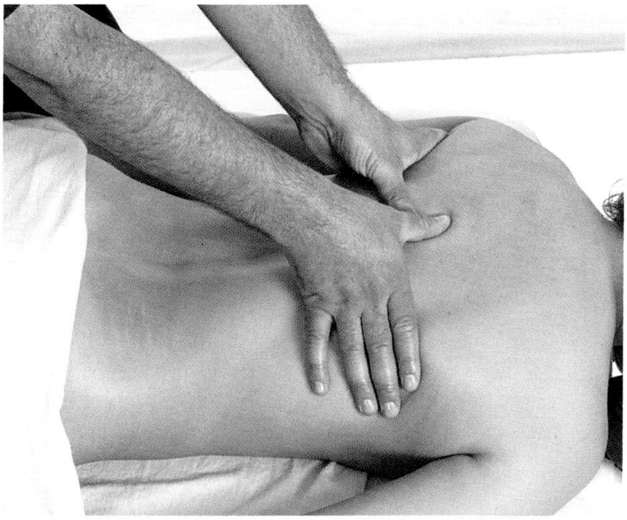

FIGURE 16-3 ■

KYPHOSIS ROUTINE

8 Using static pressure, find and deactivate all active trigger points on the middle and lower trapezius muscles.
9 Thumb-strip the lamina groove from C7 to T12.
10 Perform thumb-stripping and cross-fiber friction to the rhomboid muscles. If any active trigger points are found, deactivate them using static finger pressure (Figure 16-4).

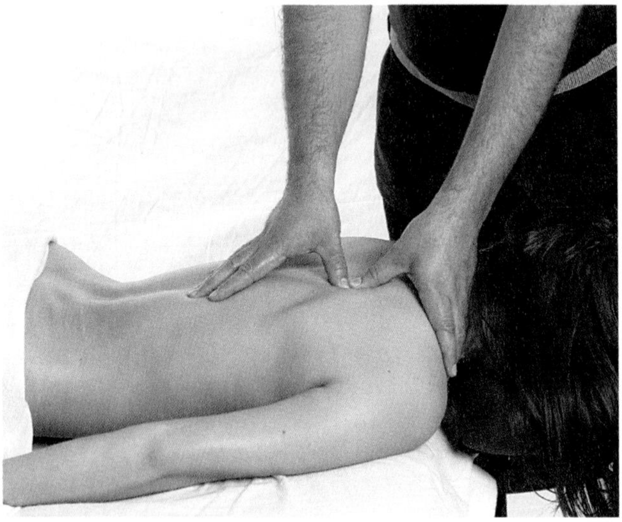

FIGURE 16-4 ■

POSITION: CLIENT IS NOW SUPINE

PROCEDURE:

1 Position the client's head over hands and use cross-fiber friction (with fingertips) on the occipital region.
2 Find and deactivate any active trigger points in the occipital ridge.
3 Holding the client's head with one hand, thumb-strip with the other hand the posterior cervical muscles along the lamina groove (Figure 16-5).

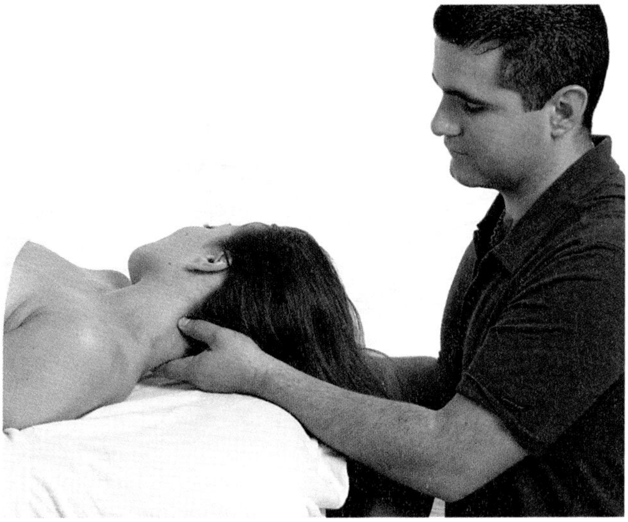

FIGURE 16-5 ■

4 Pincer-grip and uncoil the upper trapezius from the neck toward the shoulder (Figure 16-6).

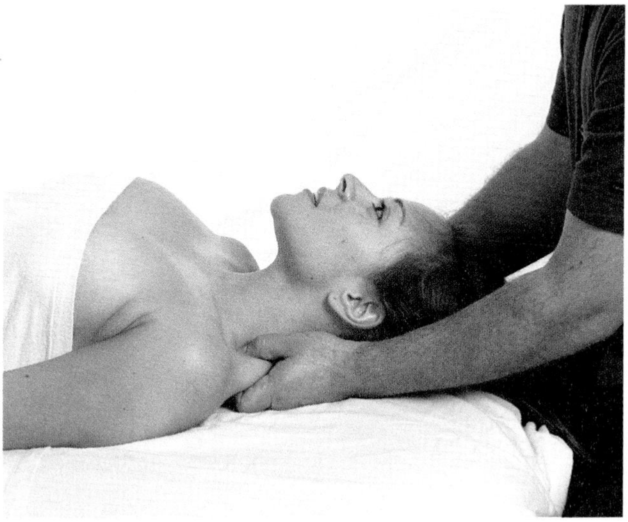

FIGURE 16-6 ■

KYPHOSIS ROUTINE

5 Find and deactivate all active trigger points on the levator scapula (especially where the neck meets the shoulder).

6 Apply effleurage and myofascial release (MFR) to the pectoralis major. To increase working area, have female clients hold breasts down if need be (Figure 16-7).

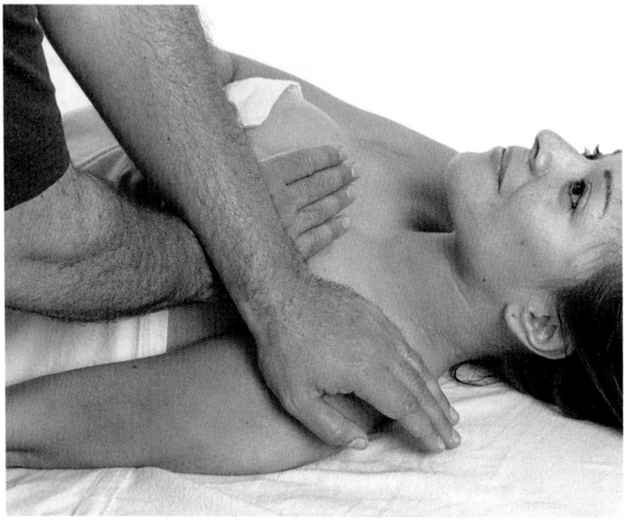

FIGURE 16-7 ■

7 Pincer-grip the pectoralis minor until pain subsides (move toward insertion) (Figure 16-8).

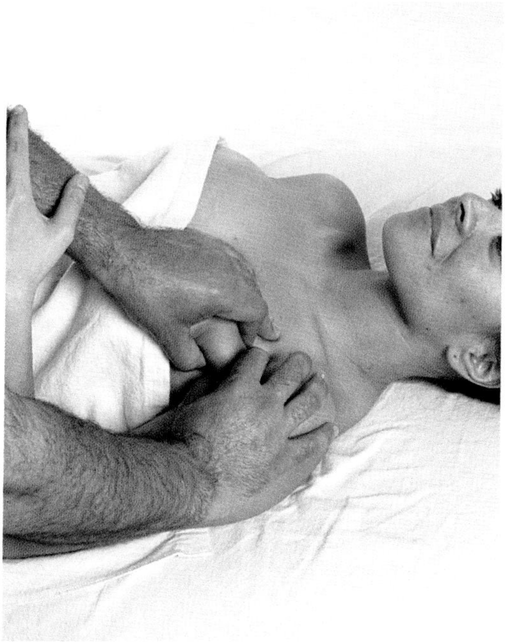

FIGURE 16-8 ■

8 Perform trigger point therapy below the origin of the pectoralis minor (coracoid process) followed by cross-fiber friction.
9 Apply with-fiber friction to the pectoralis minor (Figure 16-9).

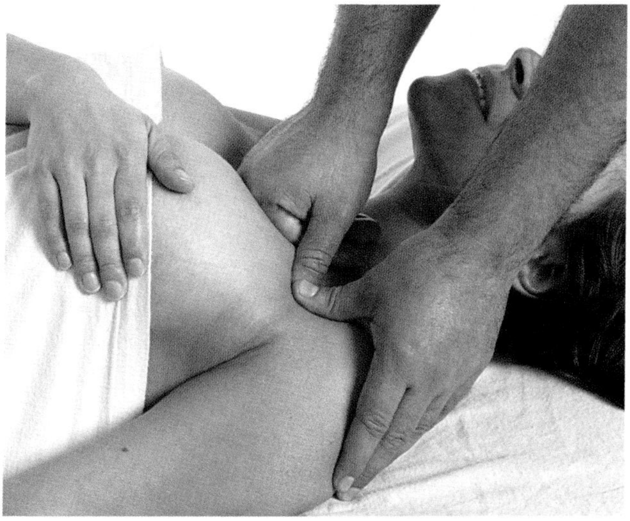

FIGURE 16-9 ■

10 Apply effleurage and perform concluding strokes to the area.
11 Stretch pectoralis muscles.

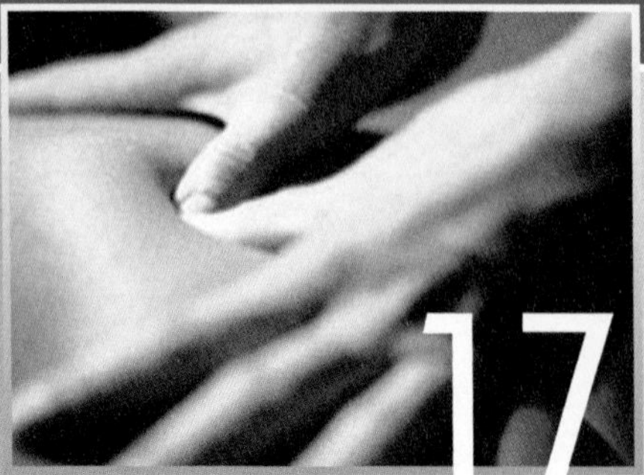

CHAPTER 17

SCOLIOSIS

OUTLINE

Definition and symptoms
Indications
Contraindications
Scoliosis routine

KEY TERMS

Scoliosis
Nonstructural scoliosis
Transient structural scoliosis
Structural scoliosis
Lumbago

OBJECTIVES

Upon completion of this chapter the reader will have the information necessary to:

1 **Define common scoliosis causes**
2 **Describe common scoliosis symptoms**
3 **Identify common scoliosis routine indications**
4 **Classify common scoliosis routine contraindications**
5 **Understand and perform a scoliosis routine**

DEFINITION AND SYMPTOMS

Scoliosis is a complicated deformity that is characterized by both lateral (side-to-side) curvature and vertebral rotation (torque) of the spine. If the disease is progressive, the vertebrae and spinous processes in the area of the major curve rotate toward the concavity of the deviation. On the concave side of the curve, the ribs rest closely together. On the convex side, they are more separated. The most common types of scoliosis are:

- **Nonstructural scoliosis**
- **Transient structural scoliosis**
- **Structural scoliosis** (approximately 80% of all cases)

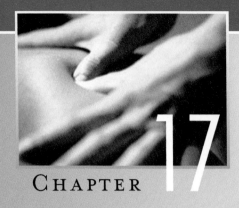

Indications

- Back pain **(lumbago)**
- Excessive side-to-side spinal curvature
- Radiating pain
- Headaches
- Migraines
- Postural misalignments

Contraindications

- Severely herniated discs
- Nerve damage
- Heart conditions
- History of stroke
- Rheumatoid arthritis
- Brittle bone disease

POSITION: CLIENT IS STANDING

PROCEDURE:

1 Compare height level of client's left and right shoulders, head tilt, anterior superior iliac spine (ASIS), knees, and ankles.
2 Observe client in standing position and compare anterior superior iliac spine (ASIS), posterior superior iliac spine (PSIS), spinal curvatures, head tilt, and spinal torque in all body planes (Figures 17-1, 17-2, 17-3, 17-4, 17-5).

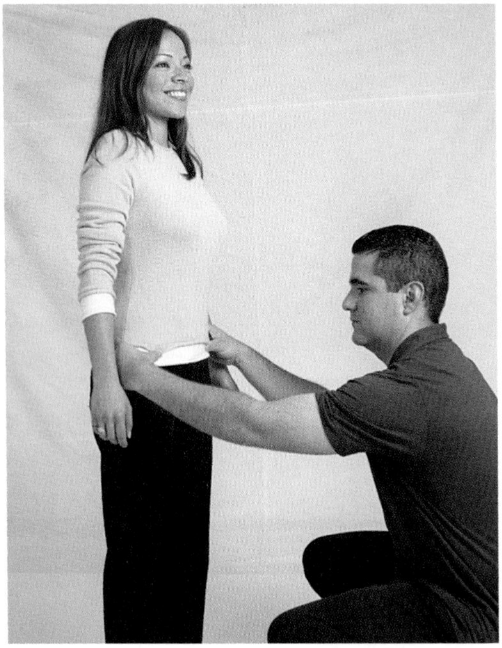

FIGURE 17-1 ■ Analyze posture by comparing height level at ASIS.

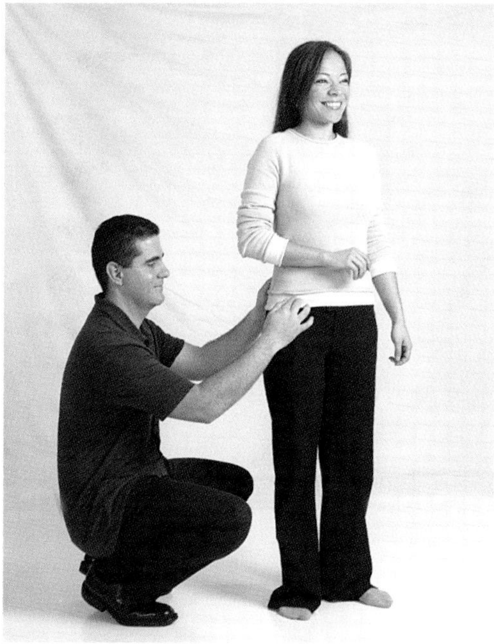

FIGURE 17-2 ■ Analyze posture by comparing level of angle between the PSIS and ASIS.

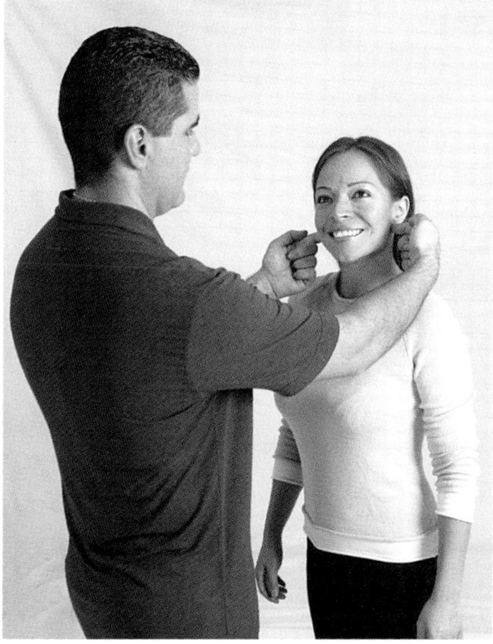

FIGURE 17-3 ■ Analyze posture by comparing height level of mastoid process.

SCOLIOSIS ROUTINE

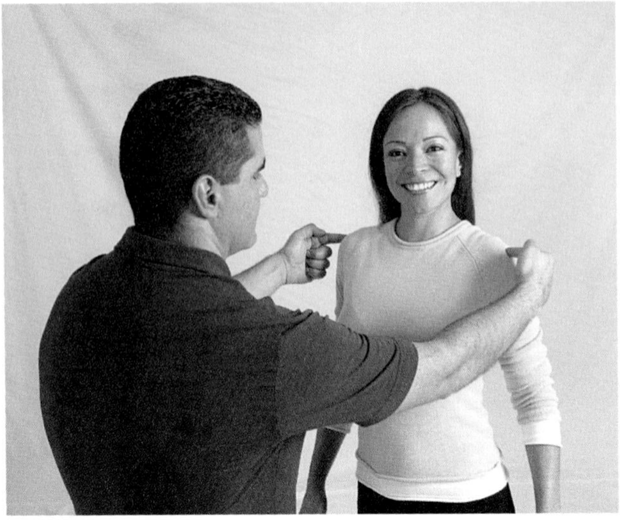

FIGURE 17-4 ■ Analyze posture by comparing height level on left and right shoulders.

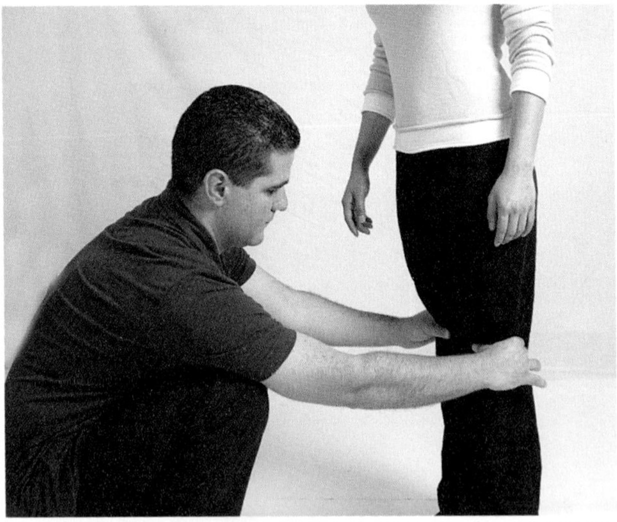

FIGURE 17-5 ■ Analyze posture by comparing height level on knees.

POSITION: CLIENT IS PRONE

PROCEDURE:

1 Effleurage and warm up the lower back area.
2 Thumb-glide and muscle-sculpt the area between the iliac crest and rib #12 (twice) (Figures 17-6 and 17-7).

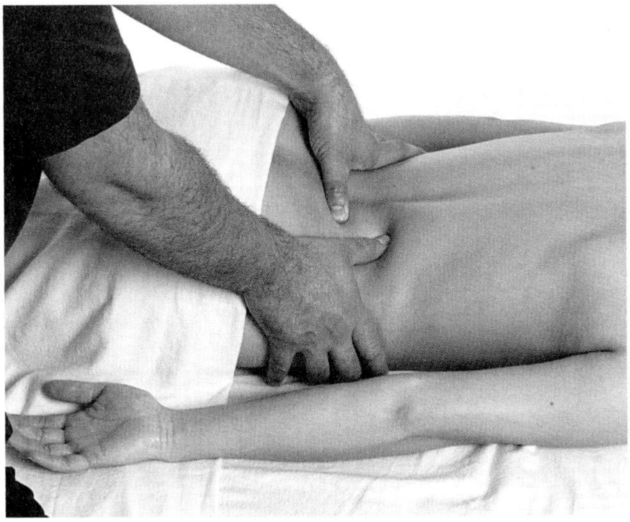

FIGURE 17-6 ■ Thumb-glide the area between the iliac crest and rib #12.

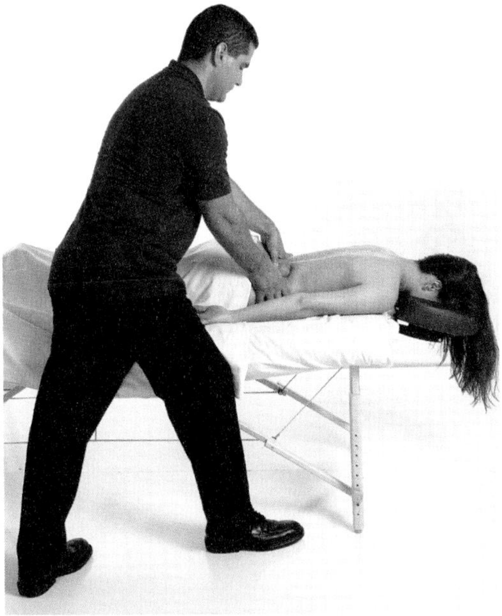

FIGURE 17-7 ■ Muscle-sculpt the area between the iliac crest and rib #12.

SCOLIOSIS ROUTINE

3 Skin-roll the entire lower back region.
4 Check the quadratus lumborum for trigger points and deactivate any active ones (Figure 17-8).
5 Perform circular friction along the spine, inferior to superior, making sure to work the affected area twice and the non-affected area once.

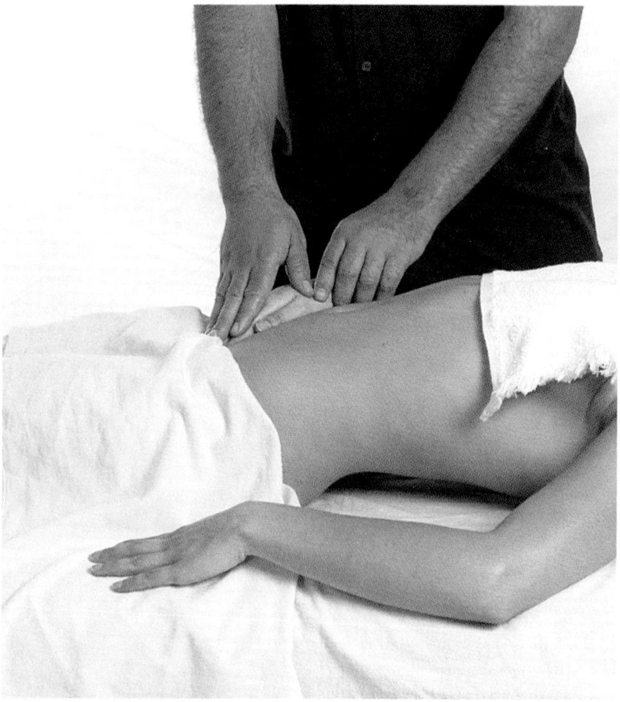

FIGURE 17-8 ■

6 Use circular and cross-fiber friction on the erector spinae (Figures 17-9 and 17-10).

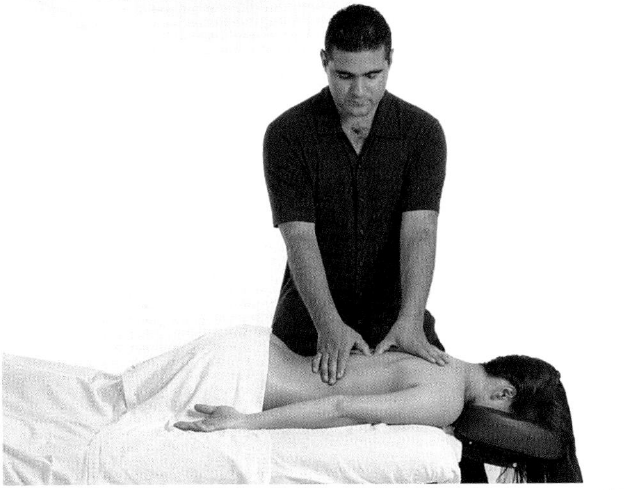

FIGURE 17-9 ■ Circular and cross-fiber friction the erector spinae (wide view).

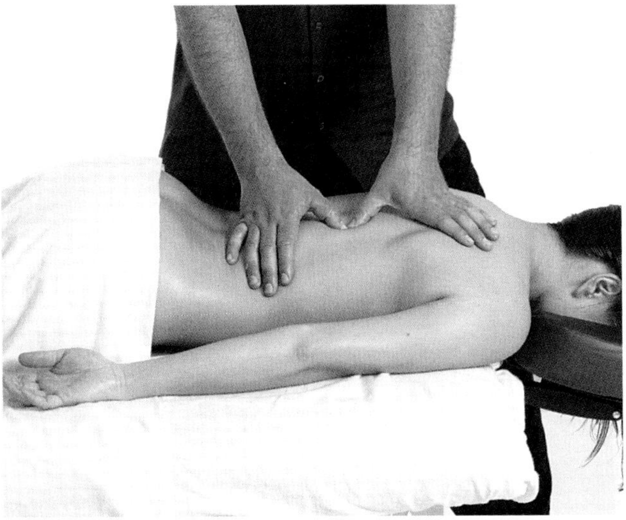

FIGURE 17-10 ■ Circular and cross-fiber friction the erector spinae (close-up view).

7 With the forearm, glide superiorly to inferiorly the whole length of the back (Figures 17-11 and 17-12).

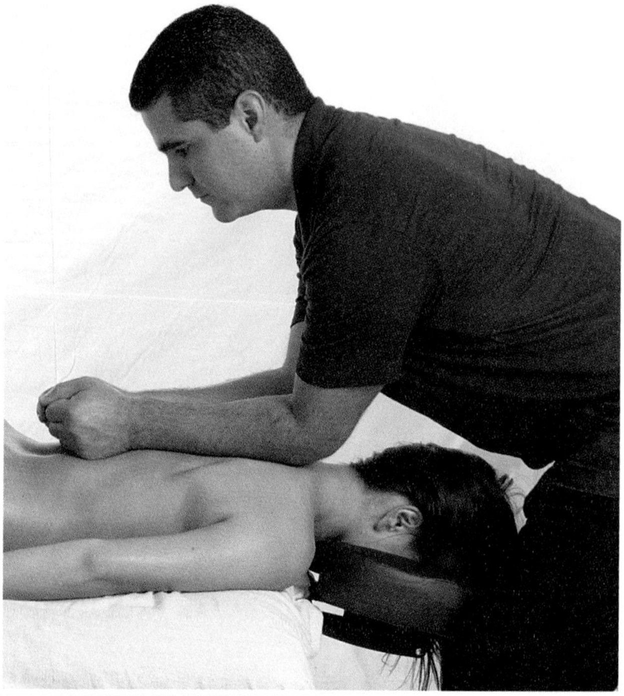

FIGURE 17-11 ■ Follow the body mechanics shown in this picture to glide superiorly to inferior with the forearm the whole length of the back.

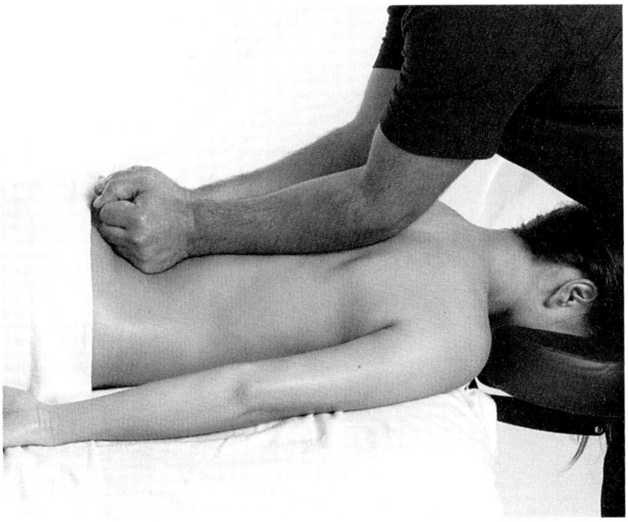

FIGURE 17-12

8 Move laterally and repeat steps 6 and 7 on the iliocostalis.
9 Muscle-sculpt and strip the rhomboids major and minor (Figures 17-13 and 17-14).

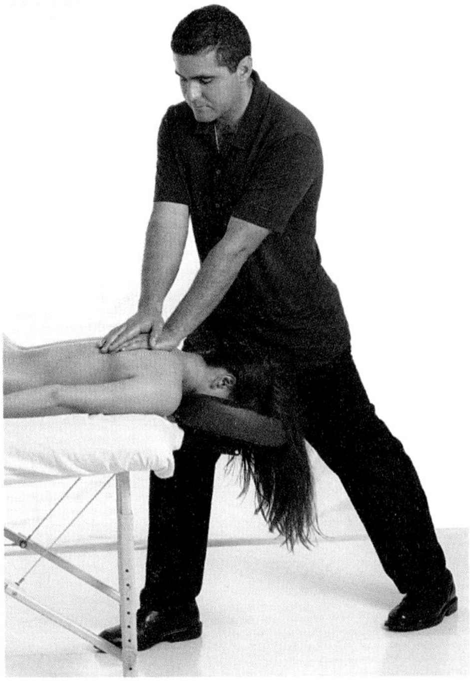

FIGURE 17-13 ■ Proper body mechanics for muscle sculpting and stripping of the rhomboids major and minor.

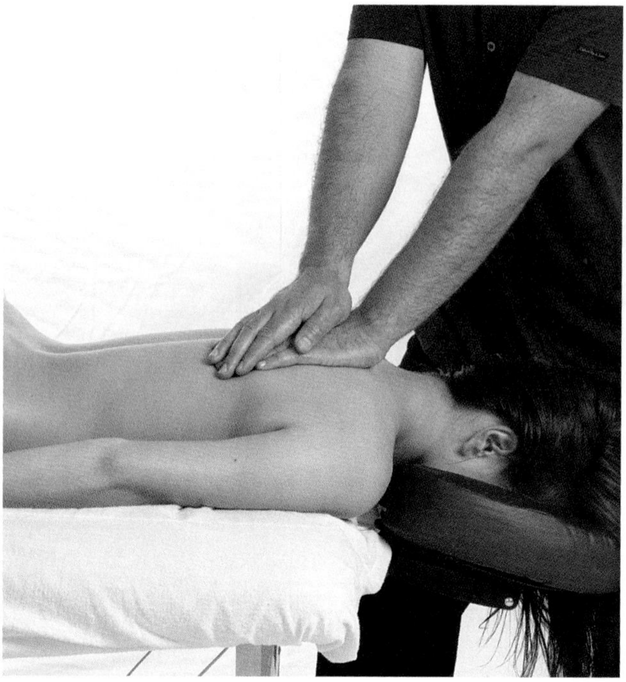

FIGURE 17-14 ■ Proper hand placement for muscle sculpting and stripping of the rhomboids major and minor.

10 Repeat steps 4 through 10 on the opposite side of the back.

POSITION: CLIENT IS SIDE-LYING

PROCEDURE:

NOTE: The following techniques are performed on the concave side only.

1 Support knee with a bolster or pillow to take the traction out of the working muscle.

2 Thumb-glide and finger-strip the transverse, internal, and exterior oblique muscles.

3 Work the origin (ribs) of the serratus anterior muscle with circular and cross-fiber friction (Figure 17-15).

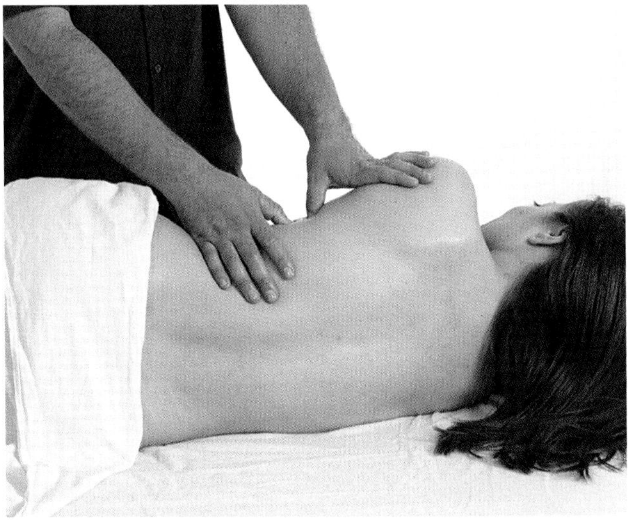

FIGURE 17-15

SCOLIOSIS ROUTINE

4 Retract the scapula, insert fingers under the vertebral border of the scapula and use cross-fiber friction right under the edge (Figures 17-16 and 17-17).

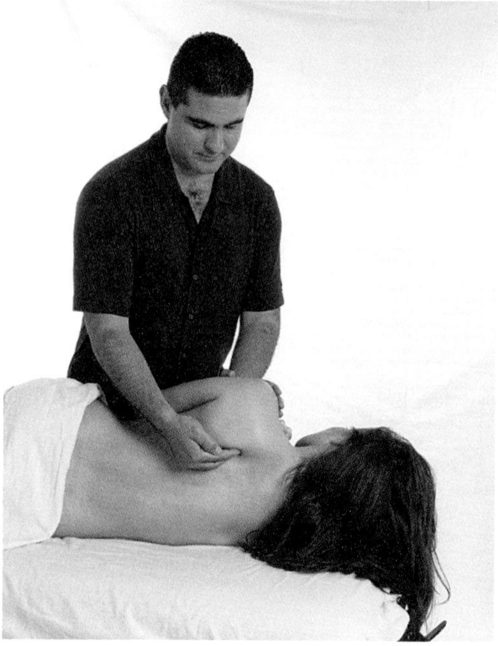

FIGURE 17-16 ■ Proper body mechanics for retracting the scapula and inserting fingers under the vertebral border of the scapula.

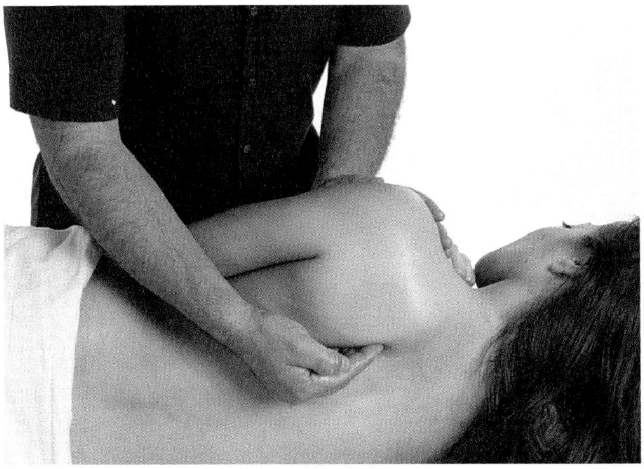

FIGURE 17-17 ■ Proper hand placement for retracting the scapula and inserting fingers under the vertebral border of the scapula.

5 Complete the treatment with effleurage and stretching of the muscles worked.

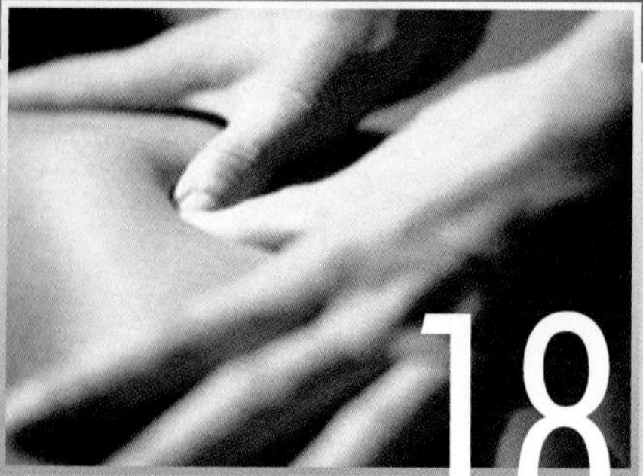

CHAPTER 18

LORDOSIS

OUTLINE

Definition and symptoms
Indications
Contraindications
Lordosis routine

KEY TERMS

Lordosis
Achondroplasia
Discitis
Kyphosis
Obesity
Osteoporosis
Spondylolisthesis

OBJECTIVES

Upon completion of this chapter the reader will have the information necessary to:

1 **Define common lordosis causes**
2 **Describe common lordosis symptoms**
3 **Identify common lordosis routine indications**
4 **Classify common lordosis routine contraindications**
5 **Understand and perform a lordosis routine**

DEFINITION AND SYMPTOMS

Lordosis is an abnormal anterior convex curvature of the lumbar spine (swayback). Lordosis (lor-doe-sis) can also be found in the neck (cervical), but it is most common in the lumbar region. A lumbar lordosis can be painful, sometimes affecting movement, posture, spinal integrity, and internal organs. It can be caused by poor posture but can also be affected by the following conditions:

- **Achondroplasia**–an inherited bone growth disorder that may cause dwarfism.
- **Discitis**–an inflammation of intervertebral disc space.
- **Kyphosis** (e.g., humpback)–may force the lower back to compensate for the imbalance created by a curve occurring at a higher level of the spine (e.g., thoracic).

- **Obesity**–may cause some overweight people to lean backward to improve balance, thereby creating an exaggerated lordotic curvature.
- **Osteoporosis**–a bone density disease that may cause vertebrae to lose strength, compromising the spine's structural integrity.
- **Spondylolisthesis** (slipped vertebrae)–occurs when one vertebra slips forward in relation to an adjacent vertebra, usually in the lumbar spine.

Indications

- Obesity
- Poor ergonomics
- Back pain
- Postural imbalance
- Exaggerated anterior pelvic tilt
- Muscle spasms

Contraindications

- Severely herniated discs
- Edema
- Acute strains
- Acute sprains

LORDOSIS ROUTINE

POSITION: CLIENT IS STANDING

PROCEDURE:

Measure the angle of the pelvis on the coronal plane (comparing the anterior superior iliac spine [ASIS] and anterior inferior iliac spine [AIIS]) and check the angle of the pelvic tilt. Average male pelvic tilt is 0 to 5 degrees; average female pelvic tilt is 5 to 10 degrees (Figure 18-1).

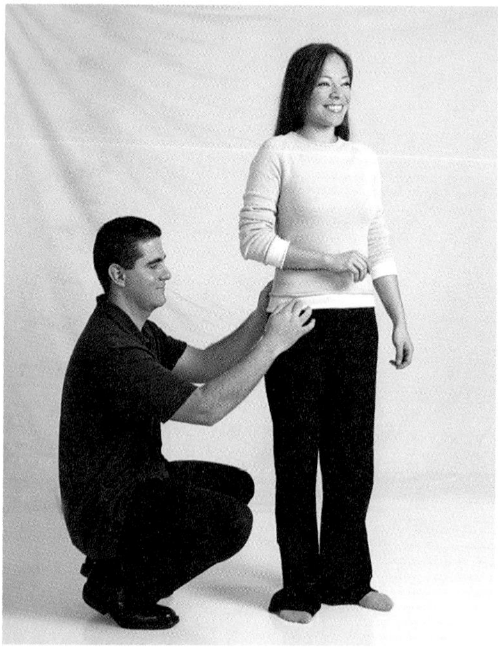

FIGURE 18-1 ■

POSITION: CLIENT IS NOW SUPINE

PROCEDURE:

1 Stretch the client's lower back muscles by bringing knees to the chest (first one and then both knees).
2 Perform pelvic stabilization by placing hands over client's ASIS, fingers on iliac crest, and perform a rocking motion side-to-side in an effort to improve pelvic height difference. Make sure to pull the correct hip down (Figures 18-2 and 18-3).

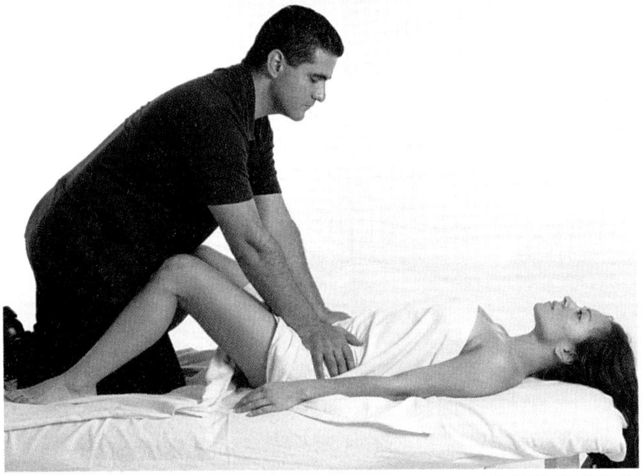

FIGURE 18-2 ■ Perform pelvic stabilization by placing hands over client's ASIS, fingers on iliac crest, and perform a rocking motion side to side in an effort to improve pelvic height difference.

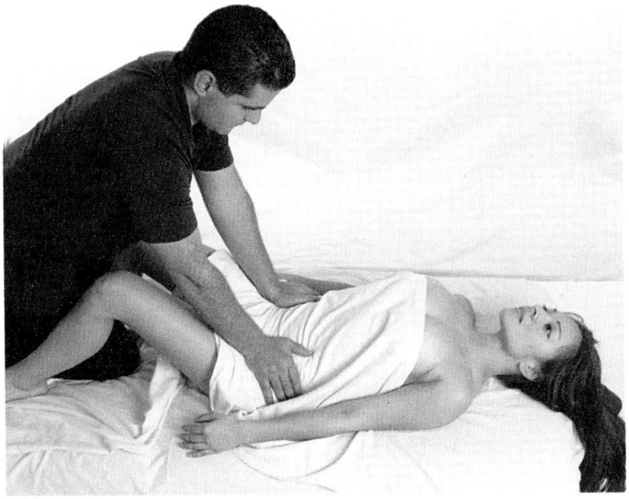

FIGURE 18-3 ■ Make sure to pull the correct hip down while performing this procedure.

LORDOSIS ROUTINE

3 Massage the rectus abdominis.

Do not work if client has an abdominal aneurysm.

4 Use cross-fiber friction on the pubic symphysis, rib attachments 5 through 7, and lateral surface of the xyphoid process (Figure 18-4).

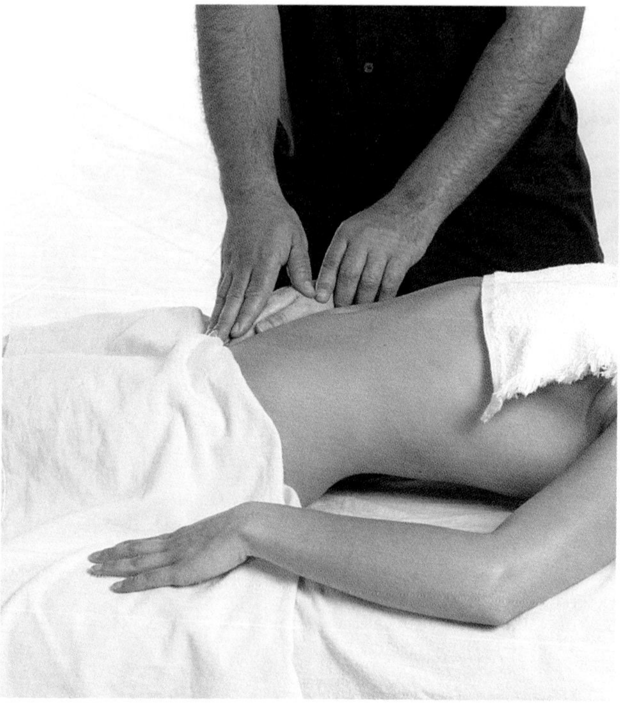

FIGURE 18-4

5 Glide across the rectus abdominis superior to inferior.
6 Massage the rest of the abdominal muscles (Figure 18-5).

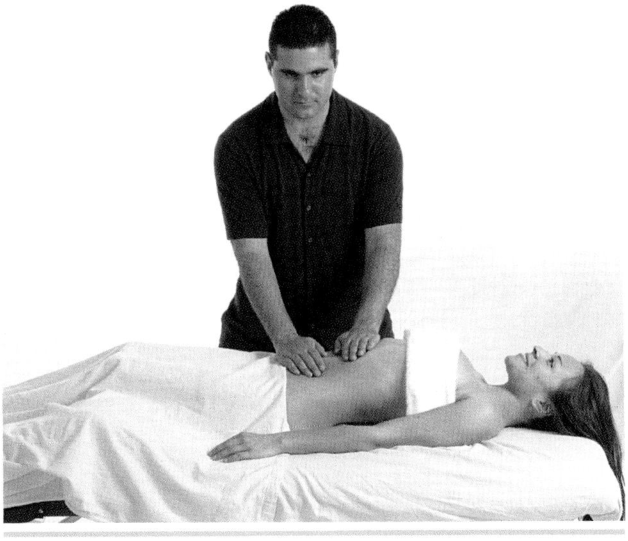

FIGURE 18-5

7 Use cross-fiber friction on ribs 5 through 12 and the iliac crest, flowing from anterior to posterior (Figure 18-6).

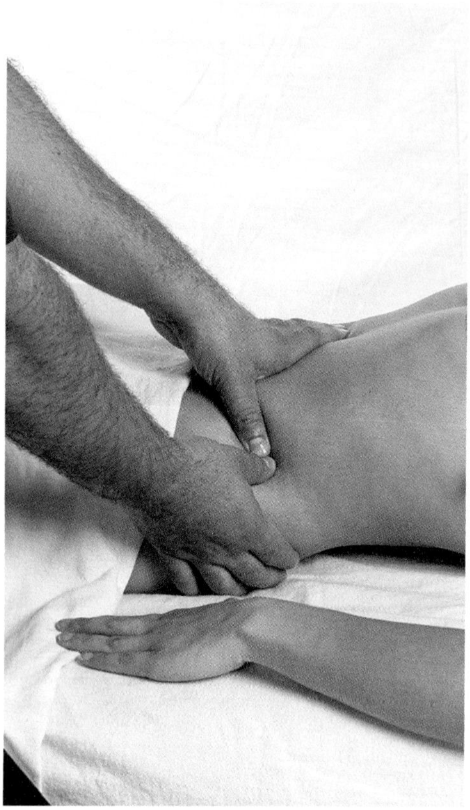

FIGURE 18-6

8 Insert fingers or thumb under the rib cage while the client exhales and use cross-fiber friction just under the ridge (Figure 18-7).

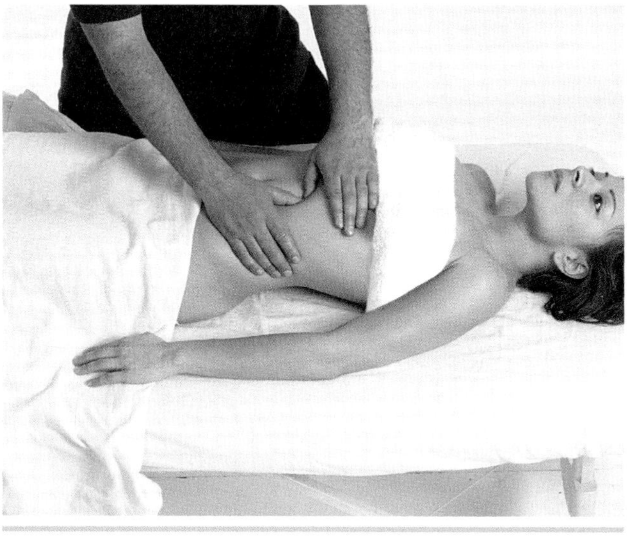

FIGURE 18-7 ■

LORDOSIS ROUTINE

9 Flex the knee (same side being worked on) to relax the iliopsoas muscle.

10 At approximately three finger widths away from the navel, begin rotating fingers clockwise to reach the psoas muscle (Figure 18-8).

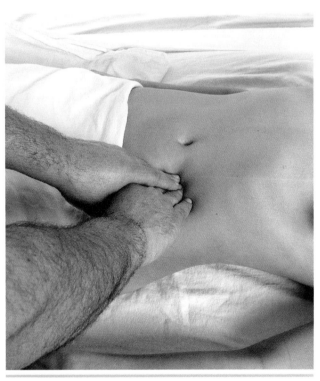

FIGURE 18-8

11 Treat the psoas insertion (lesser trochanter) with circular friction (Figure 18-9).

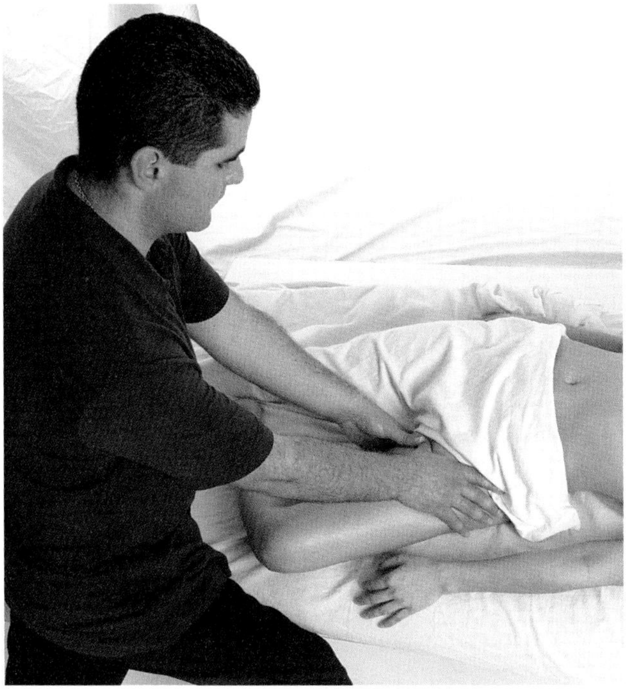

FIGURE 18-9

POSITION: CLIENT IS NOW SIDE-LYING

PROCEDURE:

1 Effleurage the iliotibial band from insertion to origin (Figure 18-10).

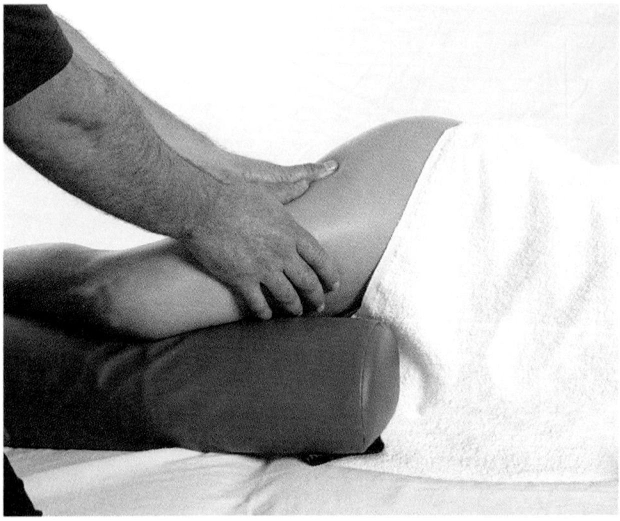

FIGURE 18-10 ■

2 Use cross-fiber friction underneath the band (Figure 18-11).

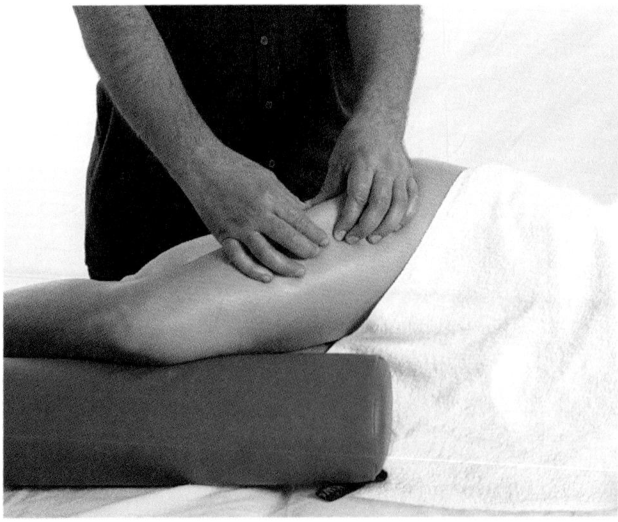

FIGURE 18-11 ■

3 Strip the belly of the tensor fasciae latae (TFL) and use cross-fiber friction on the origin and insertions (Figure 18-12).

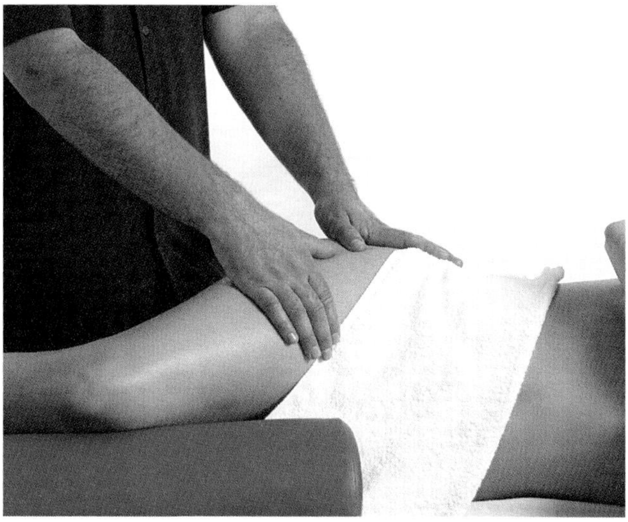

FIGURE 18-12

4 Perform advanced trunk rotation (Figure 18-13).

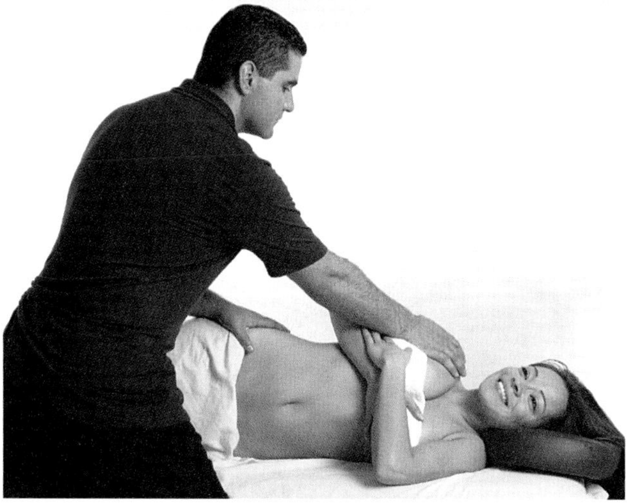

FIGURE 18-13

POSITION: CLIENT IS NOW PRONE

PROCEDURE:

1 Effleurage the entire lower back.

NOTE: A hot pack may be used to warm up the area.

2 Proceed with cross-fiber friction on the transverse processes of L1-L4.

3 Use circular and cross-fiber friction of the posterior iliac crest (Figure 18-14).

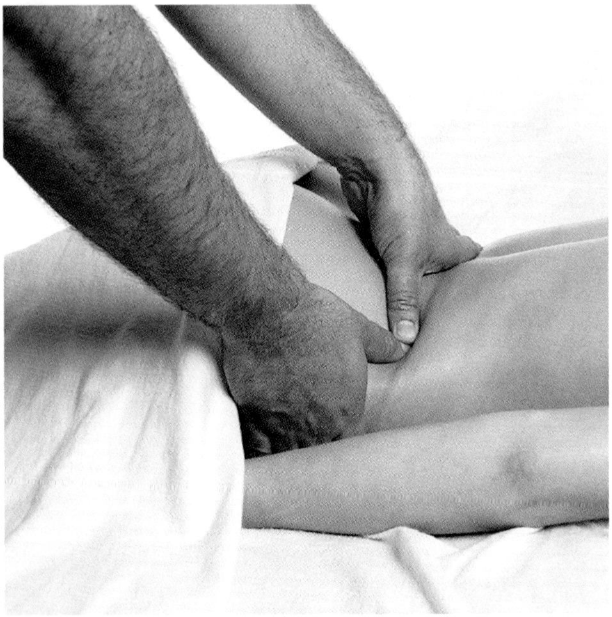

FIGURE 18-14 ■

LORDOSIS ROUTINE

4 Effleurage the erector spinae.
5 Glide on the erector spinae group using the forearm (Figure 18-15).

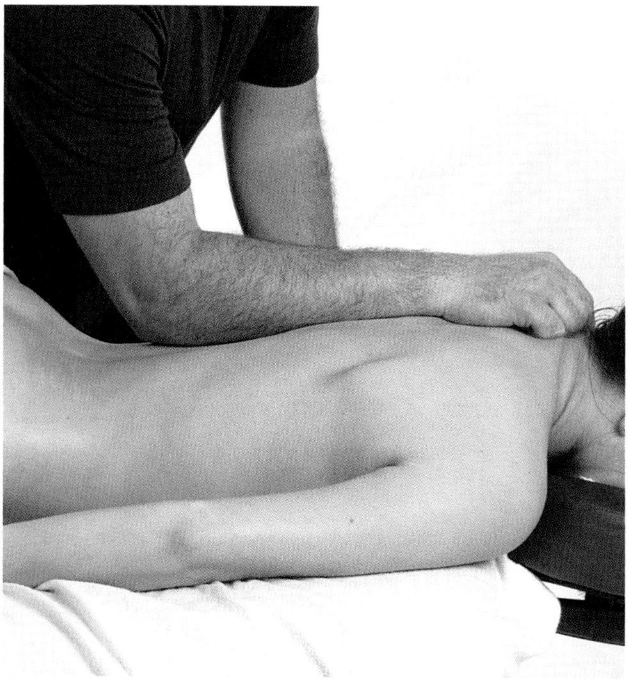

FIGURE 18-15

6 Treat the lamina groove area with circular and cross-fiber friction.
7 Perform deep effleurage from superior to inferior.
8 Perform concluding strokes.

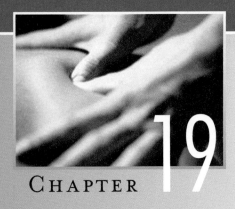

CHAPTER 19

LOWER BACK PAIN

OUTLINE

Definition and symptoms
Indications
Contraindications
Lower back pain routine

KEY TERMS

Irritated nerve roots
Spinal nerve irritation
Erector spinae strain
Cauda equina syndrome

OBJECTIVES

Upon completion of this chapter the reader will have the information necessary to:

1 **Define common lower back pain causes**
2 **Describe common lower back pain symptoms**
3 **Identify common lower back pain routine indications**
4 **Classify common lower back pain routine contraindications**
5 **Understand and perform a lower back pain routine**

DEFINITION AND SYMPTOMS

In the United States, lower back pain is one of the most common conditions affecting the population, and it is one of the leading causes of physician visits. It is estimated that at least four of every five adults will experience lower back pain at some point in his or her life.

Often the severity of the pain is unrelated to the extent of physical damage because muscle spasms, even from a simple back strain, might cause excruciating back pain that could make it difficult for a person to walk or even stand. Conversely, a large herniated or degenerated disc might be completely painless.

Icon represents an area where extreme caution should be used to avoid damage or compression to underlying or neighboring vessels.

Symptoms can be aggravated by the following:

- **Irritated nerve roots**
- **Spinal nerve irritation**
- **Erector spinae strain**
- Injured bones, ligaments, or joints
- Injured intervertebral disc
- Menstrual cramping

There are several symptoms that are possible indications of a serious medical condition, and clients with these symptoms should seek medical attention immediately:

- Sudden bowel and/or bladder incontinence **(cauda equina syndrome)**
- Progressive weakness in the legs (cauda equina syndrome)
- Severe, continuous abdominal and back pain
- Fever and chills
- History of cancer with recent weight loss
- Acute severe trauma

Indications

- Lower back spasms
- Radiating pain down legs
- Reduced range of motion (ROM)
- Poor posture
- Muscle strains

Contraindications

- History of cancer
- Kidney infection
- Acute severe trauma
- Severe abdominal pain
- Leg weakness
- Edema

POSITION: CLIENT IS STANDING

PROCEDURE:

Measure the angle of the pelvis on the coronal plane (comparing the anterior superior iliac spine [ASIS] and posterior superior iliac spine [PSIS]) and check the angle of the pelvic tilt. Average male pelvic tilt is 0 to 5 degrees; average female pelvic tilt is 5 to 10 degrees (Figure 19-1).

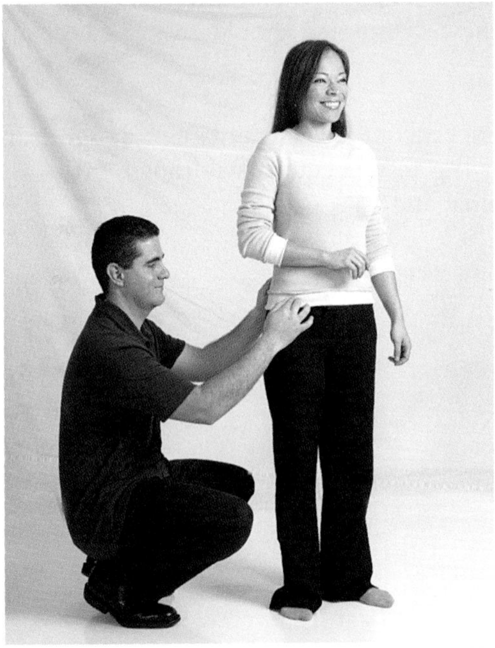

FIGURE 19-1 ■

POSITION: CLIENT IS NOW SUPINE

PROCEDURE:

1 Stretch the lower back muscles by bringing knees to the chest (first one and then both knees).
2 Perform pelvic stabilization by placing hands over client's ASIS, fingers on iliac crest, and perform a rocking motion side to side in an effort to improve pelvic height difference. Make sure to pull the correct hip down (Figures 19-2 and 19-3).

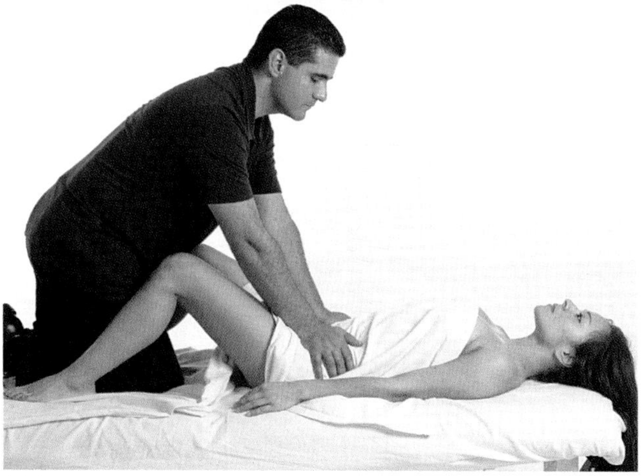

FIGURE 19-2 ■ Perform pelvic stabilization by placing hands over client's ASIS, fingers on iliac crest, and perform a rocking motion side to side in an effort to improve pelvic height difference.

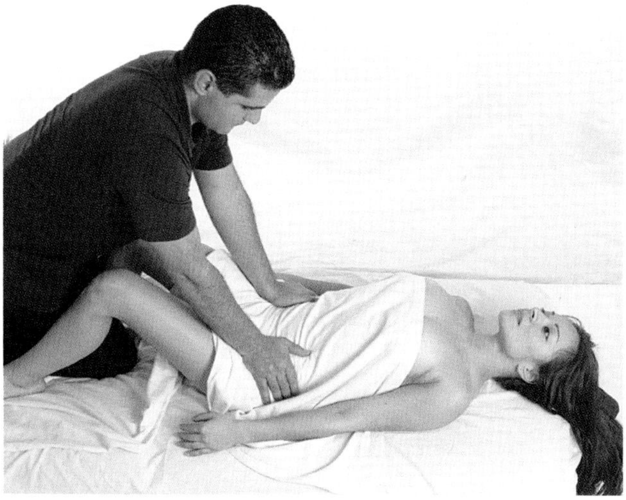

FIGURE 19-3 ■ Make sure to pull the correct hip down while performing this procedure.

3 Massage the rectus abdominis (Figures 19-4).

⚠ *Do not work if client has abdominal aneurysm(s).*

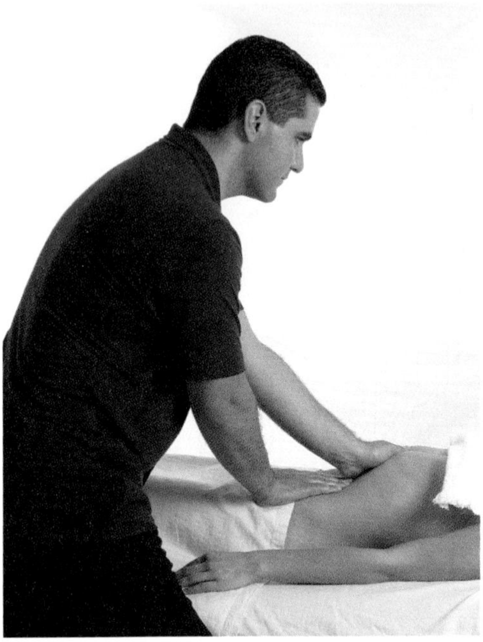

FIGURE 19-4

4 Use cross-fiber pubic symphysis, rib attachments 5 through 7, and lateral surface of the xyphoid process (Figure 19-5).

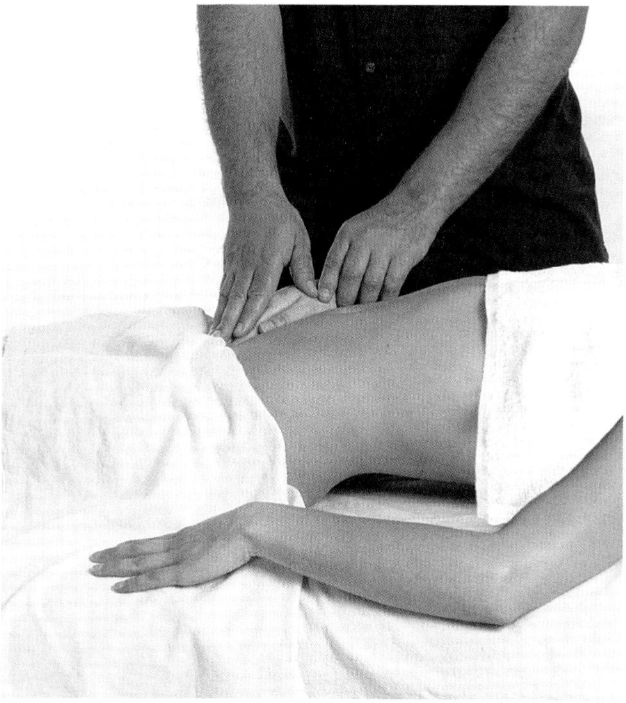

FIGURE 19-5

5 Glide across the rectus abdominis superior to inferior.
6 Massage the rest of the abdominal muscles.
7 Use cross-fiber friction on ribs 5 through 12 and the iliac crest, flowing from anterior to posterior.

8 Insert fingers or thumb under the rib cage while client exhales and use cross-fiber friction just under the ridge (Figure 19-6).

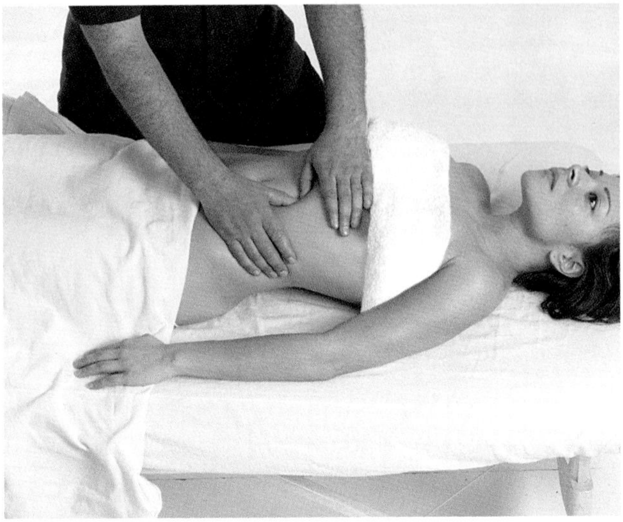

FIGURE 19-6 ■

9 Flex the knee to relax the iliopsoas muscle (Figure 19-7).

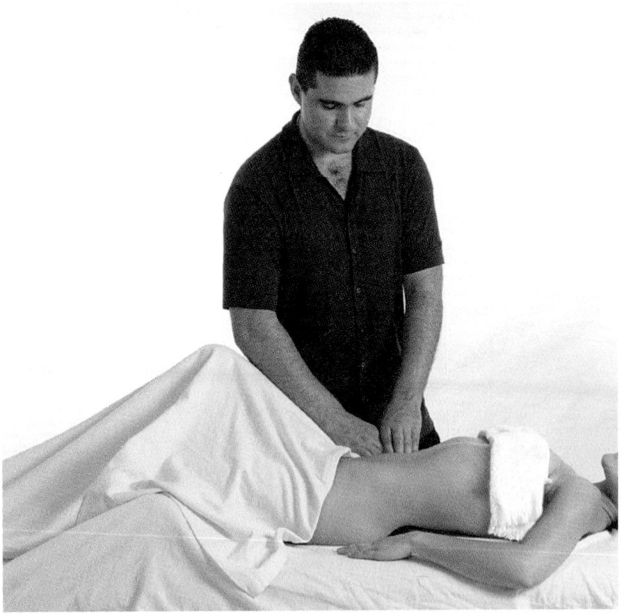

FIGURE 19-7 ■

LOWER BACK PAIN ROUTINE

10 Approximately three finger widths away from the navel begin rotating fingers clockwise to reach the psoas muscle (Figure 19-8). Treat the psoas insertion (lesser trochanter) with circular friction.

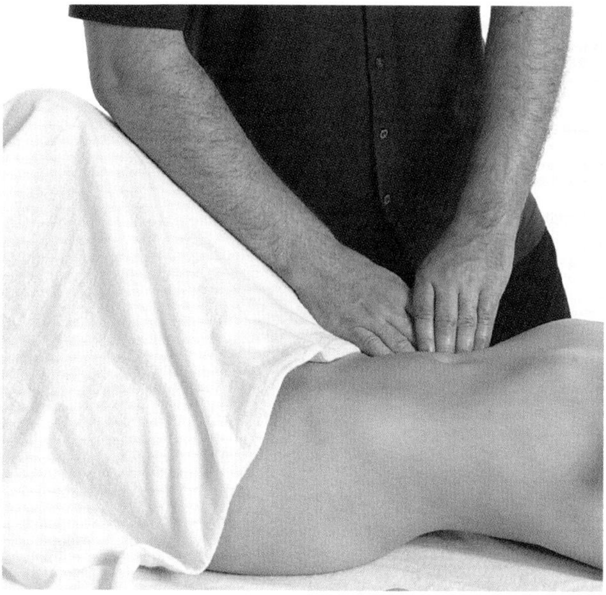

FIGURE 19-8 ■

POSITION: CLIENT IS NOW SIDE-LYING

PROCEDURE:

1 Effleurage the iliotibial band from insertion to origin.
2 Use cross-fiber friction underneath the band (Figure 19-9).

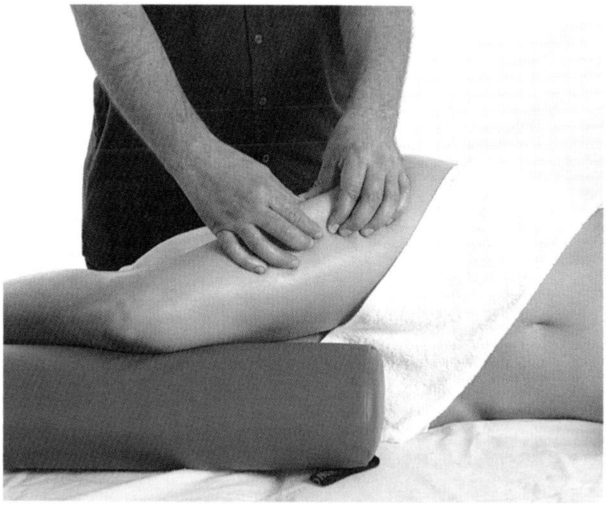

FIGURE 19-9 ■

LOWER BACK PAIN ROUTINE

3 Strip the belly of the tensor fascia latae and use cross-fiber friction on the origin and insertions (Figure 19-10).

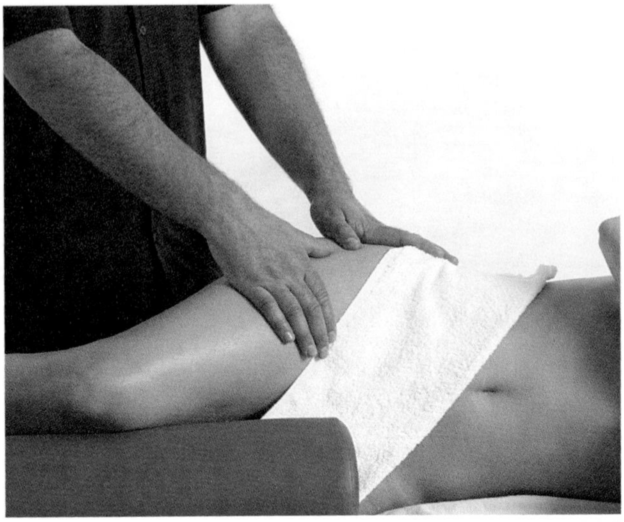

FIGURE 19-10

POSITION: CLIENT IS NOW PRONE

PROCEDURE:

1 Effleurage the entire lower back

NOTE: Hot pack may be used to warm up the area.

2 Proceed with cross-fiber friction on the transverse processes of L1-L4 (Figure 19-11).

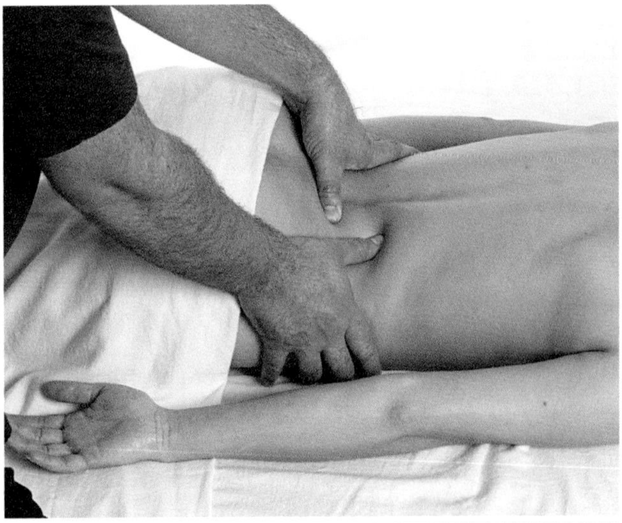

FIGURE 19-11

3 Use circular and cross-fiber friction on the posterior iliac crest.
4 Effleurage the erector spinae.
5 Glide the erector spinae group using the forearm (Figure 19-12).

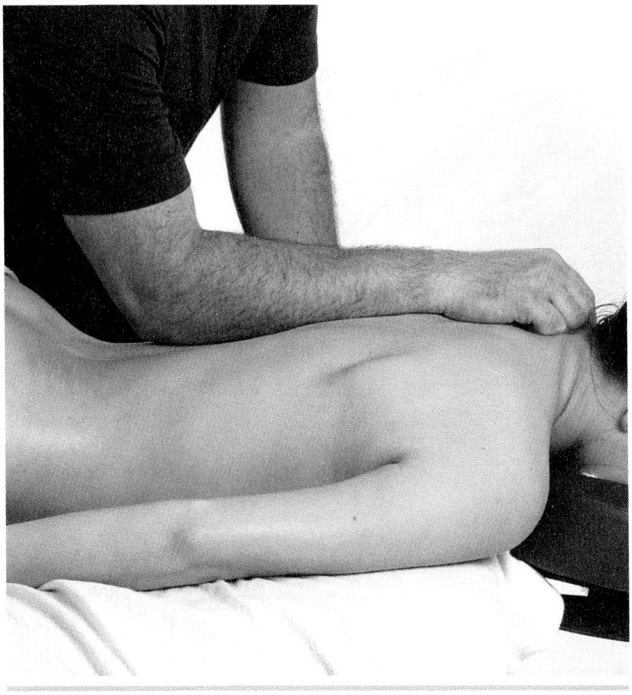

FIGURE 19-12

6 Treat the lamina groove area with circular and cross-fiber friction.
7 Perform deep effleurage from superior to inferior and back.
8 Perform concluding strokes.

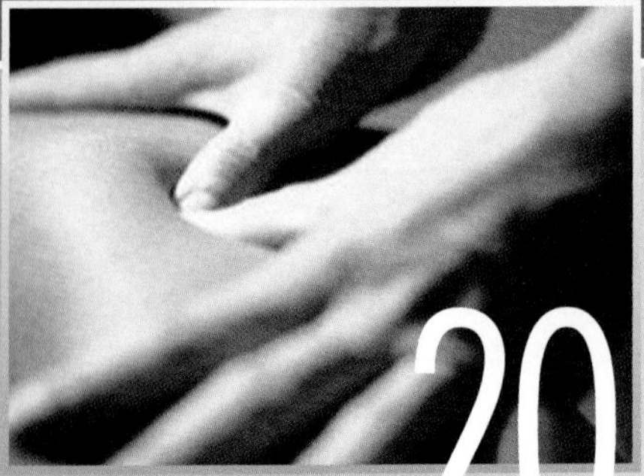

CHAPTER 20

ILIOPSOAS DISORDER

OUTLINE

Definition and symptoms
Indications
Contraindications
Iliopsoas disorder routine

KEY TERMS

Iliopsoas
Spondylolysis
Spondylolisthesis

OBJECTIVES

Upon completion of this chapter the reader will have the information necessary to:

1. **Define common iliopsoas disorder causes**
2. **Describe common iliopsoas disorder symptoms**
3. **Identify common iliopsoas disorder routine indications**
4. **Classify common iliopsoas disorder routine contraindications**
5. **Understand and perform a iliopsoas disorder routine**

DEFINITION AND SYMPTOMS

The **iliopsoas** is the most important active postural or stabilizing muscle of the hip joint, and a hip flexor. Studies have shown that the iliopsoas made up for paralyzed abductor muscles when it was attached to the greater trochanter, proving that stability to the pelvis was more important than the reduction of hip flexor power. Any weakening or shortening of the iliopsoas will most likely result in lower back pain.

The constant pull of the iliopsoas on the lumbar spine could also be related to **spondylolysis** and **spondylolisthesis**.

Indications

- Menstrual cramping
- Lower back pain (see Chapter 19)
- Lordosis (see Chapter 18)
- **Scoliosis** (see Chapter 17)
- Muscle strains

Contraindications

- History of cancer
- Abdominal lumps
- Severe abdominal pain
- Hernias
- Severe vascular disorders

ILIOPSOAS DISORDER ROUTINE

POSITION: CLIENT IS PRONE

PROCEDURE:

1 Effleurage and perform warm-up techniques on the quadratus lumborum muscle.
2 Perform myofascial release (MFR) and palm-spreading on the quadratus lumborum.
3 Use cross-fiber friction just above the iliac spine, below rib 12, and on the lamina groove.
4 Look for and deactivate trigger points in the origin, insertion, and belly of quadratus lumborum.

POSITION: CLIENT IS NOW SUPINE

PROCEDURE:

1 Warm up the abdominal area by performing a basic abdominal massage. Effleurage the external and internal oblique muscles and the transverse abdominus. Massage both sides of the body and continue by spreading along the rectus abdominus (superior to inferior and medial to lateral) (Figure 20-1).

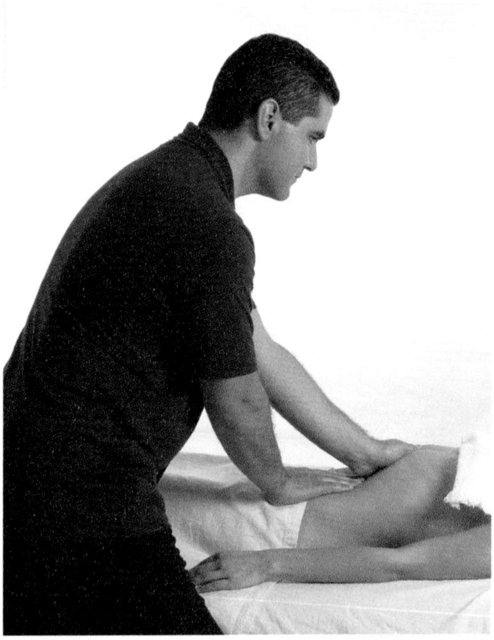

FIGURE 20-1 ■ Warm up the abdominal area by performing a basic abdominal massage.

NOTE: Always follow the direction of the large intestinal flow.

2 Start abdominal routine (in a clockwise direction) on the left side of the body. Begin deep-spreading (scooping) of the large intestine, and move from the descending colon to the transverse to the ascending colon (Figure 20-2).

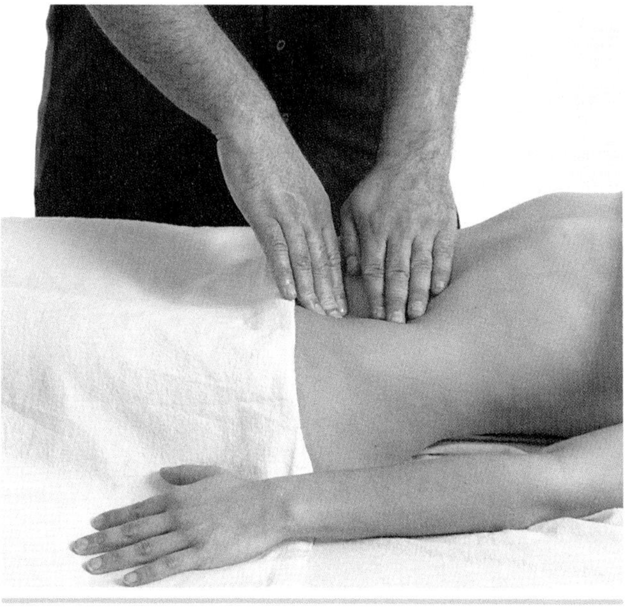

FIGURE 20-2

ILIOPSOAS DISORDER ROUTINE

3 Flex thigh on the side to be released, place elbow on the thigh, measure 2 or 3 fingers away from the navel toward the side to be released (Figures 20-3 and 20-4).

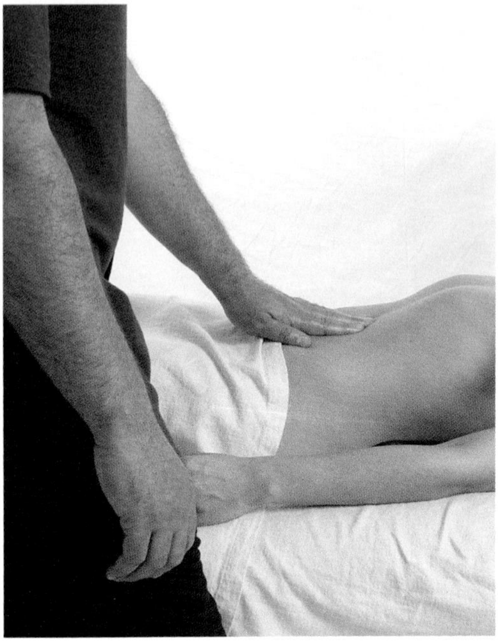

FIGURE 20-3

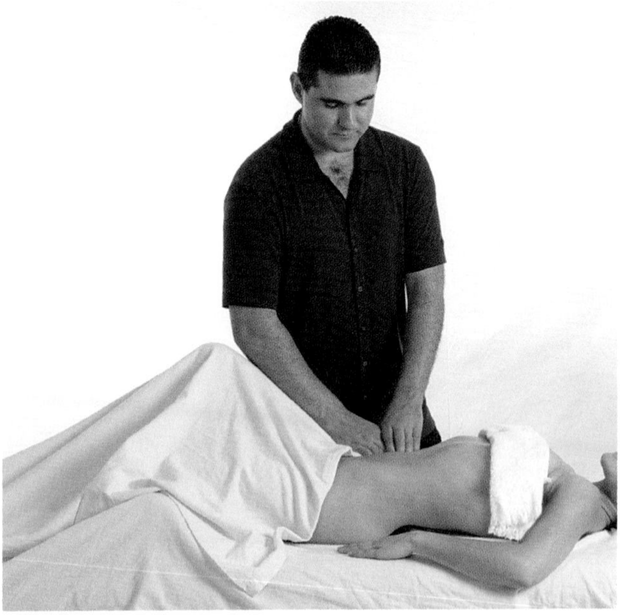

FIGURE 20-4 ■ Place elbow on the thigh—measure 2 or 3 fingers away from the navel (belly button) toward the side you will be releasing.

4 With clockwise (circular) motion, place fingertips above iliopsoas muscle and as the client exhales penetrate into the abdominal area to locate the iliopsoas muscle. Move slowly as you penetrate deeper into the abdominal region (Figure 20-5).

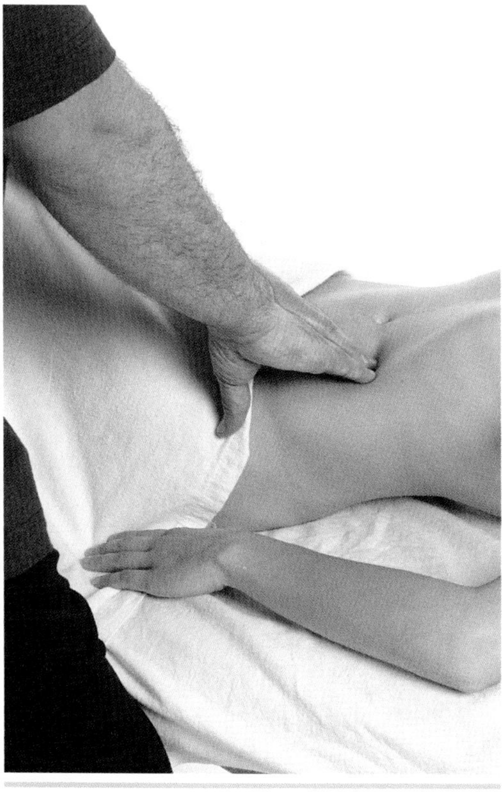

FIGURE 20-5

ILIOPSOAS DISORDER ROUTINE

5 To verify the location of the iliopsoas muscle, ask the client to resist against your elbow with their flexed knee for a few seconds until you feel the iliopsoas under your fingertips (Figures 20-6 and 20-7).

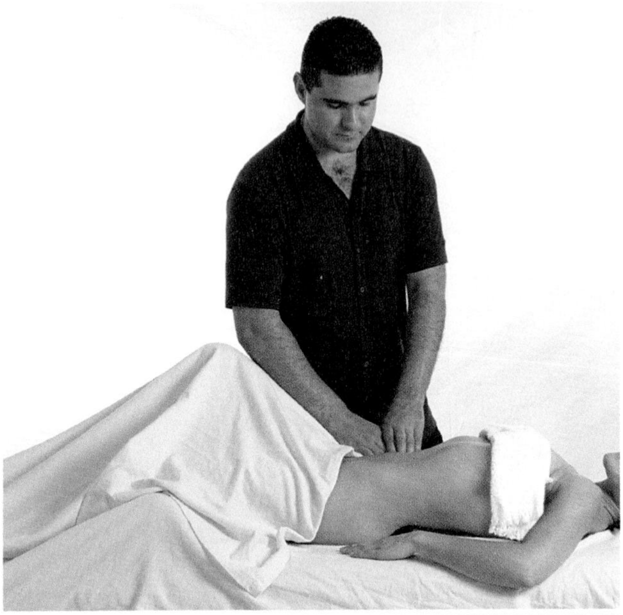

FIGURE 20-6 ■ Wide view showing how to check to make sure you are working on the psoas.

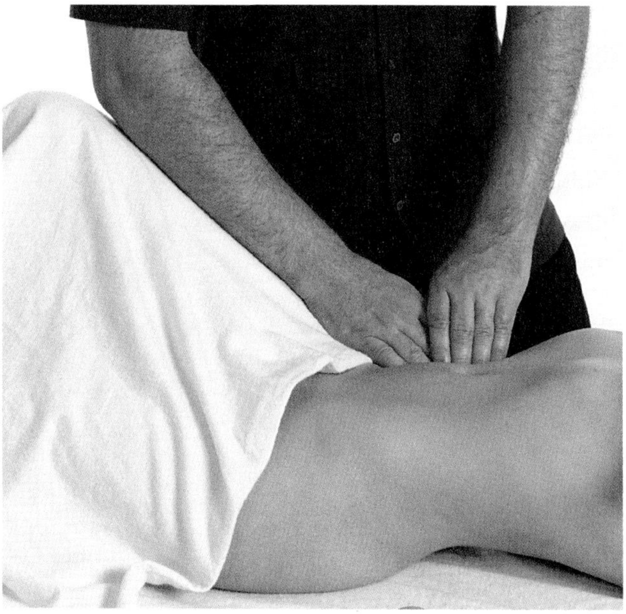

FIGURE 20-7 ■ To check if you are on the psoas—have client resist against your elbow (a few seconds only). You will feel the psoas contract under your fingertips.

6 After the iliopsoas is located, look for and deactivate trigger points and then slowly use transverse friction on the iliopsoas.
7 Remove hand gently and slowly.
8 Effleurage the area.
9 Perform stretching (while client is side-lying and supine).

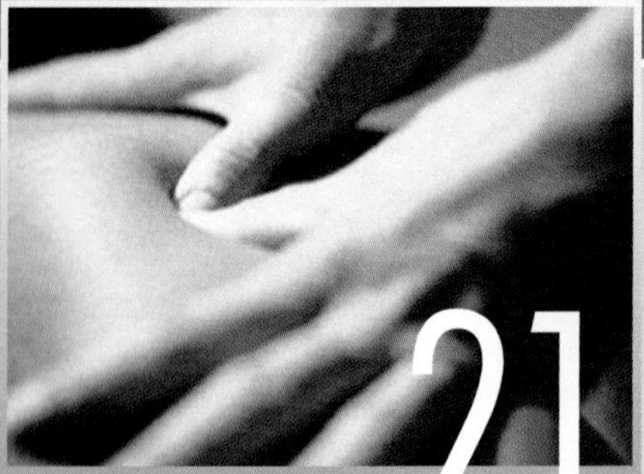

CHAPTER 21

ABDOMINAL MASSAGE (CONSTIPATION)

OUTLINE

Definition and symptoms
Indications
Contraindications
Abdominal massage (constipation)

KEY TERM

Constipation

OBJECTIVES

Upon completion of this chapter the reader will have the information necessary to:

1. **Define common constipation causes**
2. **Describe common constipation symptoms**
3. **Identify common abdominal massage (constipation) routine indications**
4. **Classify common abdominal massage (constipation) routine contraindications**
5. **Understand and perform an abdominal massage (constipation) routine**

DEFINITION AND SYMPTOMS

Constipation is an obstruction in the large intestine that prohibits the passage of stool through its normal path to the colon for elimination. Food passes through the small intestine as a liquid mixture of digestive juices and eaten food. When it reaches the large intestine, all the nutrients have been absorbed. The large intestine has one main function: to absorb water from the waste liquid and turn it into a waste solid (stool). Constipation can be caused by too much water being absorbed by the large intestine, leaving a very hard and dry stool that cannot be passed without straining. Constipation can often lead to more severe conditions such as hemorrhoids. Common factors slowing down the colon include inactivity, a diet low in fiber, not eating

Icon represents an area where extreme caution should be used to avoid damage or compression to underlying or neighboring vessels.

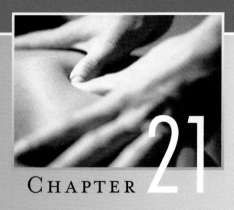

enough to stimulate the intestines to move food along, consuming certain high-protein foods, and many over-the-counter and prescription drugs.

Common causes of constipation:

- Low fluid intake. The colon absorbs enough water to prevent dehydration, resulting in less lubrication and dry, hard stools.
- Holding in bowel movements despite the urge to go. This keeps stool in the colon longer, where more water is absorbed and stool gets even harder.
- Poor diet. Not maintaining a well-balanced diet, one rich in fiber to promote bowel movements.

Indications

- Low bowel movement frequency
- Chronic constipation

Contraindications

- Severe abdominal pain
- Intestinal bleeding
- Abdominal edema
- Throbbing lump
- Strangulated hernias

ABDOMINAL MASSAGE (CONSTIPATION) ROUTINE

POSITION: CLIENT IS SUPINE

PROCEDURE:

NOTE: All strokes must be made clockwise to coincide with the direction of the large intestine.

1 Warm up the abdominal area by applying effleurage in a clockwise direction.
2 Effleurage the rectus abdominus from superior to inferior (xyphoid process to just below the navel).
3 Effleurage the external and internal oblique muscles, and transverse abdominus (Figure 21-1).

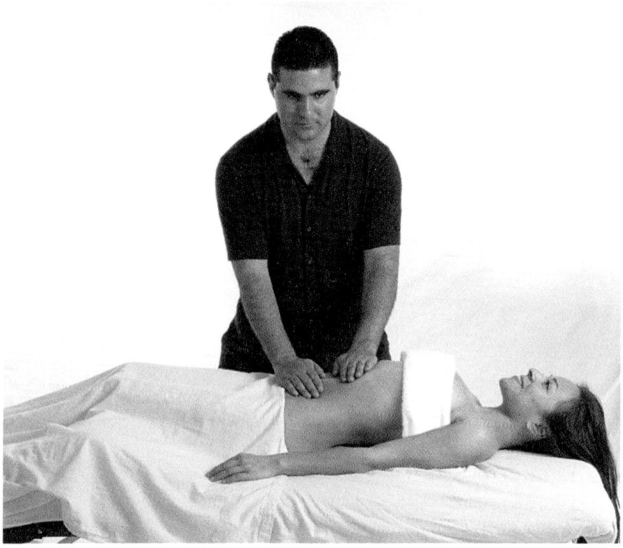

FIGURE 21-1 ■

ABDOMINAL MASSAGE (CONSTIPATION) ROUTINE

4 Once the area has been warmed up, begin scooping the end of the descending colon and scooping downward toward the sigmoid colon. Proceed with the motion heading upwards toward the transverse colon (Figure 21-2).

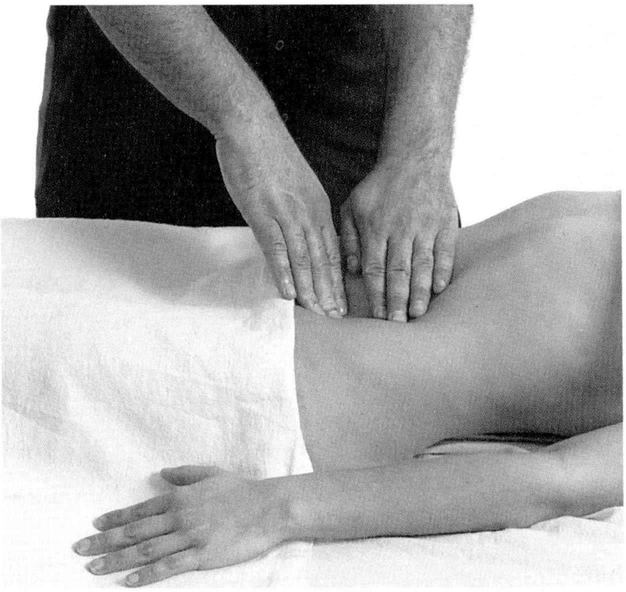

FIGURE 21-2

ABDOMINAL MASSAGE (CONSTIPATION) ROUTINE

5 Once the entire descending colon has been cleared, perform one long, deep effleurage stroke from the beginning to the end of the descending colon.

6 Repeat scooping motion for the transverse colon, making sure to begin at the descending colon junction and end at the ascending colon junction.

NOTE: Ease the pressure over the linea alba.

7 Once scooping is complete for the transverse colon, perform a deep effleurage to the descending colon (going downward), followed by a deep effleurage in an inverted L shape over the transverse and descending colon (Figure 21-3).

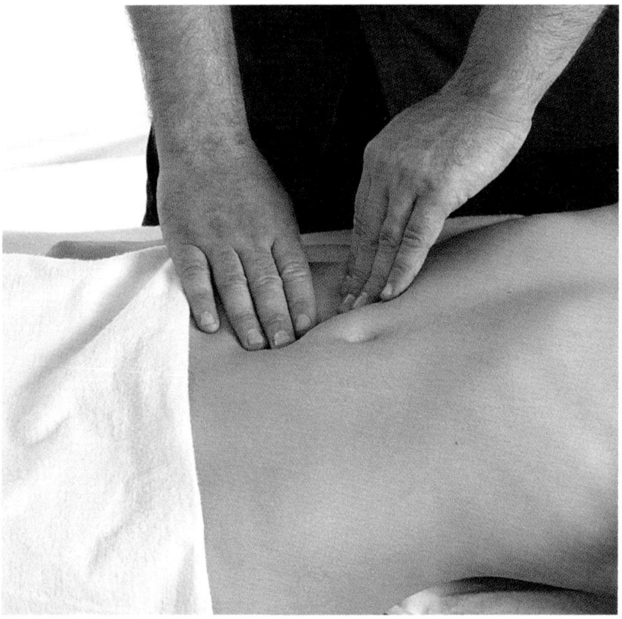

FIGURE 21-3

ABDOMINAL MASSAGE (CONSTIPATION) ROUTINE

8 Finalize by scooping the ascending colon beginning at the transverse-ascending junction heading downward (scooping toward the liver).
9 Perform a deep effleurage to the descending colon (heading downward), transverse colon (heading from right to left), and ascending colon (flowing upward).
10 Finalize treatment by performing clockwise effleurage and feather strokes.

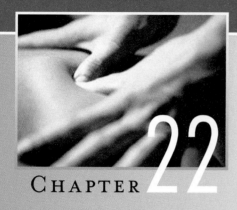

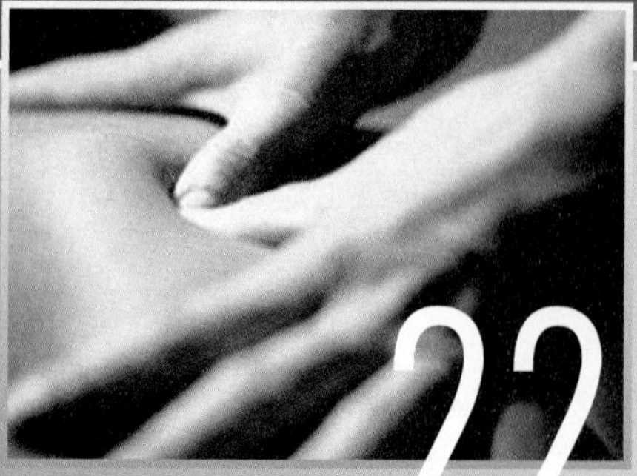

CHAPTER 22

PIRIFORMIS SYNDROME (SCIATICA)

OUTLINE

Definition and symptoms
Indications
Contraindications
Piriformis syndrome (sciatica) routine

KEY TERMS

Piriformis syndrome (sciatica)
Paresthesia

OBJECTIVES

Upon completion of this chapter the reader will have the information necessary to:

1. **Define common piriformis syndrome (sciatica) causes**
2. **Describe common piriformis syndrome (sciatica) symptoms**
3. **Identify common piriformis syndrome (sciatica) routine indications**
4. **Classify common piriformis syndrome (sciatica) routine contraindications**
5. **Understand and perform a piriformis syndrome (sciatica) routine**

DEFINITION AND SYMPTOMS

Piriformis syndrome (sciatica) is a condition in which the piriformis muscle irritates the sciatic nerve, causing pain in the buttocks and referring pain along the course of the sciatic nerve (back of the thigh). Patients generally complain of pain deep in the buttocks, which is aggravated by sitting, climbing stairs, or performing squats.

The piriformis is the first muscle of the six deep lateral rotators of the thigh, originating from the sacral spine and attaching to the greater trochanter of the femur. It assists in abducting and laterally rotating the thigh. The sciatic nerve usually passes underneath the piriformis muscle, but in 15% of individuals it travels through the muscle.

Some causes of sciatica include disease in the lumbar spine such as disc herniations, chronic hamstring tendonitis, strained piriformis, lumbago, and fibrous adhesions of other muscles around the sciatic nerve.

Indications

- Pain radiating down the buttock
- Pain radiating down posterior thigh
- Lumbago
- Muscle spasms

Contraindications

- Spinal disc edema
- Acute trauma
- Loss of movement to the affected leg
- **Paresthesia** (a burning or prickling sensation)
- Varicose veins

PIRIFORMIS SYNDROME (SCIATICA) ROUTINE

POSITION: CLIENT IS PRONE

PROCEDURE:

1 Place pillow or bolster under pelvis if lower back curvature is severe (lordosis, see Chapter 18).
2 Begin treatment by performing a basic five-minute massage to the lower back region.
3 Effleurage the hamstrings from inferior to superior.
4 Perform petrissage and deep open-fisting to the hamstrings (Figure 22-1).

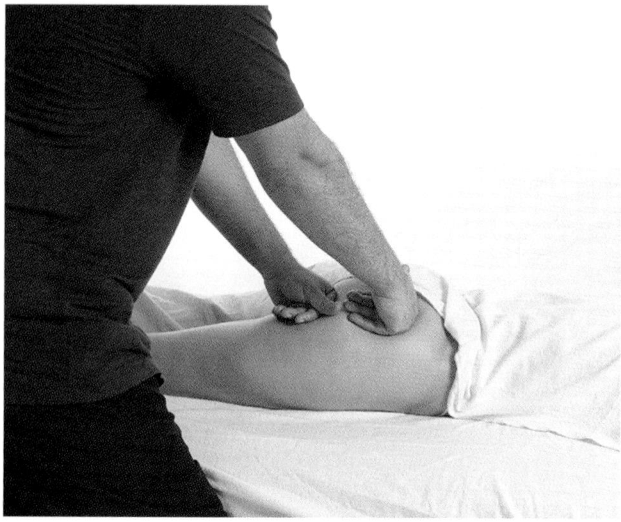

FIGURE 22-1 ■

PIRIFORMIS SYNDROME (SCIATICA) ROUTINE

5 Find the belly of the three hamstrings and thumb-strip entire area from inferior to superior (popliteal toward ischium).
6 Find and deactivate all active trigger points in the hamstring muscles.
7 To find the origin of the hamstring, place hand over leg and ask client to resist. Once found use cross-fiber friction on hamstring origin (ischial tuberosity), making sure not to use cross-fiber on bone.
8 Undrape the gluteus maximus and effleurage the entire area with open fist.
9 Perform thumb-spreading and circular-fisting on the same area (Figures 22-2 and 22-3).

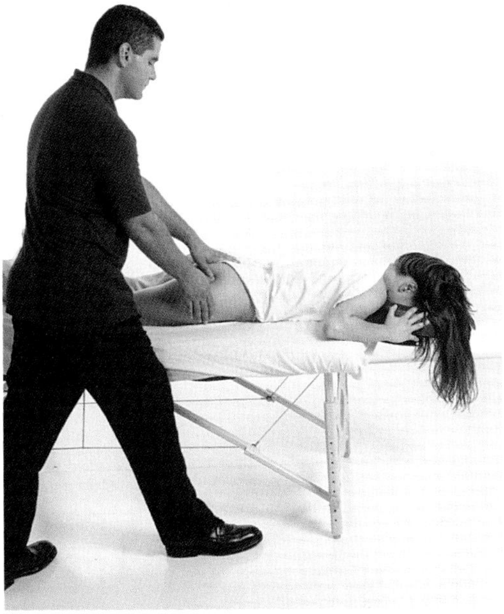

FIGURE 22-2 ■ Proper body mechanics should be observed at all times.

PIRIFORMIS SYNDROME (SCIATICA) ROUTINE

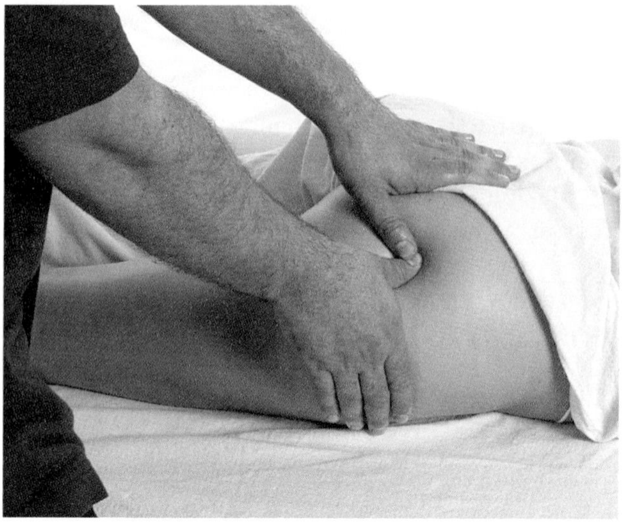

FIGURE 22-3 ■ Perform thumb-spreading.

10 Proceed up the edge of the sacrum (not on bone) with cross-fiber friction (Figure 22-4).

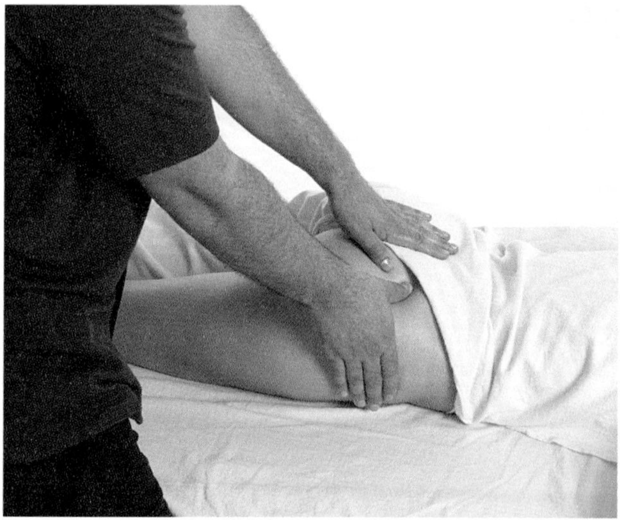

FIGURE 22-4 ■

PIRIFORMIS SYNDROME (SCIATICA) ROUTINE

11 Find and deactivate all active trigger points (not the piriformis belly because the sciatic nerve is under it). Search for trigger points on the gluteus medius. Skin-rolling may also be done at this time.

12 Begin with cross-fiber friction to the origin and insertion of the piriformis and thumb-strip the belly, being careful not to exceed patient's pain tolerance (not to exceed 8 on a 1-10 scale) (Figure 22-5).

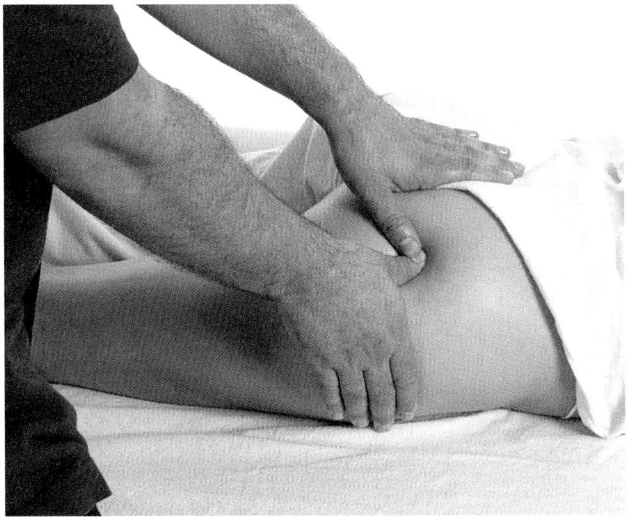

FIGURE 22-5 ■

PIRIFORMIS SYNDROME (SCIATICA) ROUTINE

13 Move knee laterally (to easily find the greater trochanter) and apply circular friction around the greater trochanter (Figure 22-6).

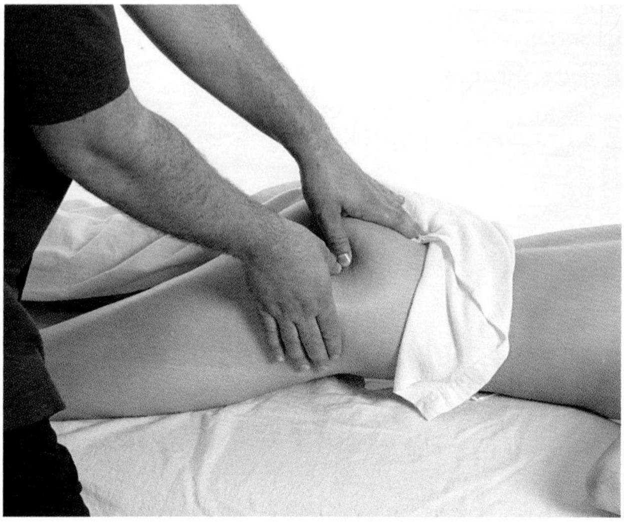

FIGURE 22-6 ■

PIRIFORMIS SYNDROME (SCIATICA) ROUTINE

14 Conclude with thumb-spreading and effleurage.
15 Cover area and perform compressions with fist below the iliac crest and above the greater trochanter.
16 Finalize treatment with stretches to the hamstrings, piriformis, and lower back.

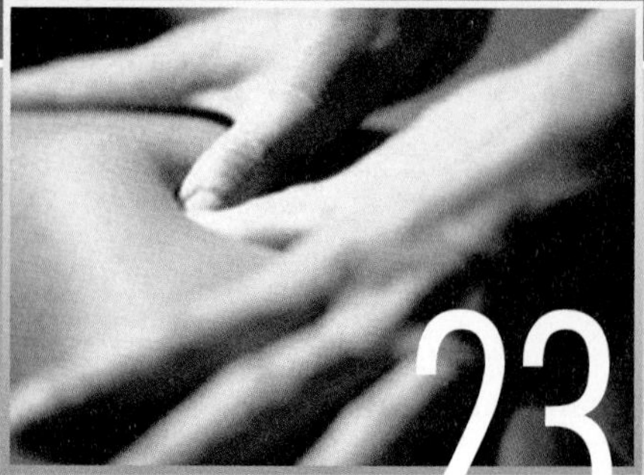

CHAPTER 23

QUADRICEPS DYSFUNCTION

OUTLINE

Definition and symptoms
Indications
Contraindications
Quadriceps dysfunction routine

KEY TERMS

Quadriceps dysfunction

OBJECTIVES

Upon completion of this chapter the reader will have the information necessary to:

1. **Define common quadriceps dysfunction causes**
2. **Describe common quadriceps dysfunction symptoms**
3. **Identify common quadriceps dysfunction routine indications**
4. **Classify common quadriceps dysfunction routine contraindications**
5. **Understand and perform a quadriceps dysfunction routine**

DEFINITION AND SYMPTOMS

Quadriceps dysfunction is a condition known to cause weakness, paresthesia, reduced knee and hip range of motion (ROM), and cramping. This dysfunction could be the result of trauma, inactivity, overuse, strains, or other thigh-related ailments. Symptoms include numbness, a tingling feeling, knee pain, and cramping. There are four muscles that compose the quadriceps group, but only one (rectus femoris) crosses the hip joint, which makes it more vulnerable to injury.

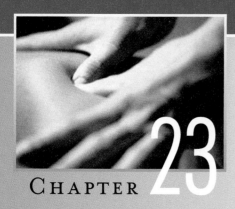

Indications

- Thigh pain
- Reduced range of motion (ROM)
- Muscle weakness
- Cramping
- Postural misalignments

Contraindications

- History of vascular disease
- Varicose veins
- Acute injury
- Edema

POSITION: CLIENT IS SUPINE

PROCEDURE:

1 Effleurage and warm up the extremity beginning at the leg and ending at the thigh.
2 Deep effleurage the quadriceps group.
3 Thumb-strip (with-fiber friction) the belly of the quadriceps group beginning just above the patella and ending two inches below the anterior superior iliac spine (ASIS) (Figure 23-1).

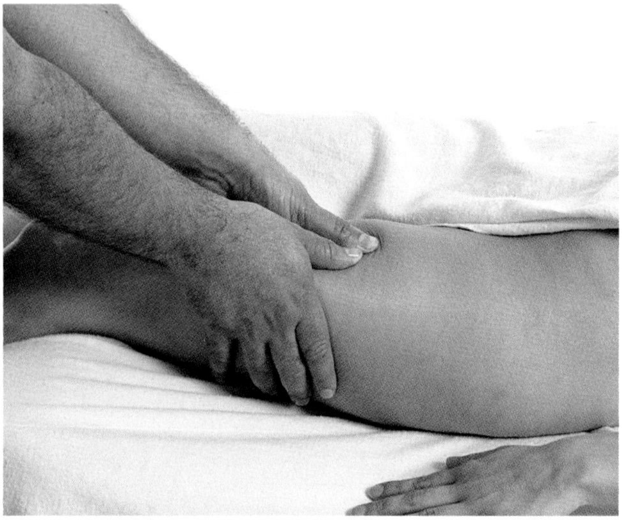

FIGURE 23-1

QUADRICEPS DYSFUNCTION ROUTINE

4 Use cross-fiber friction at the origin and insertion of the rectus femoris muscle (Figure 23-2).

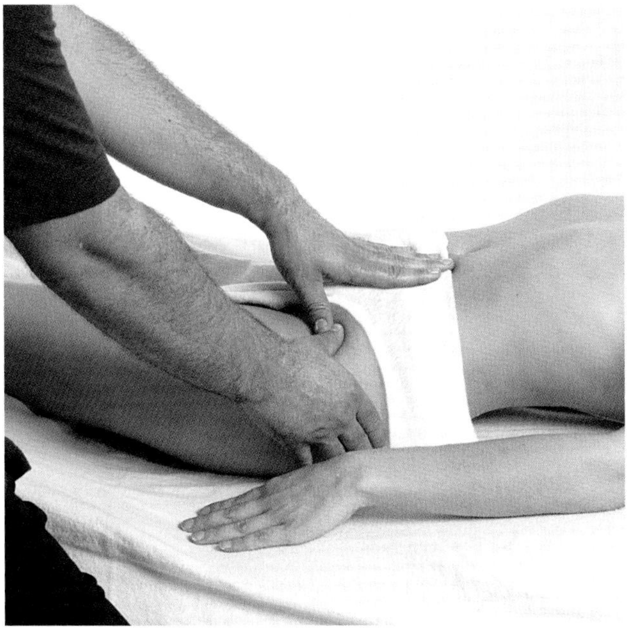

FIGURE 23-2

5 Perform circular friction around the patella (Figure 23-3).

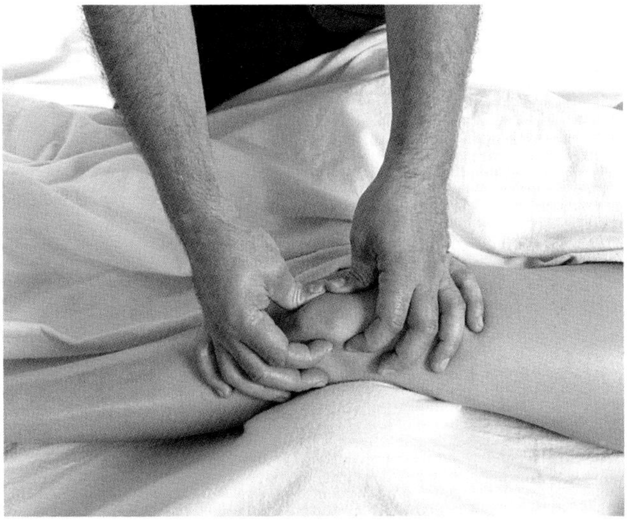

FIGURE 23-3

QUADRICEPS DYSFUNCTION ROUTINE

6 Find and deactivate all active trigger points in the quadriceps group, paying close attention to the vastus medialis and lateralis (Figure 23-4).

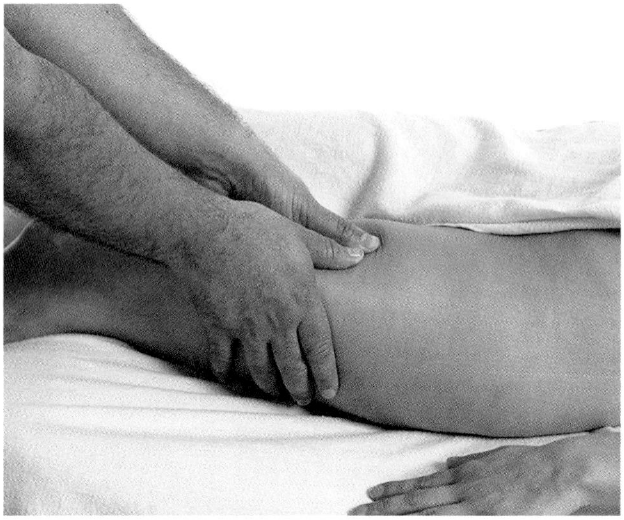

FIGURE 23-4 ■

7 Proceed with open-fist effleurage, moving up the thigh on the rectus femoris (Figures 23-5 and 23-6).

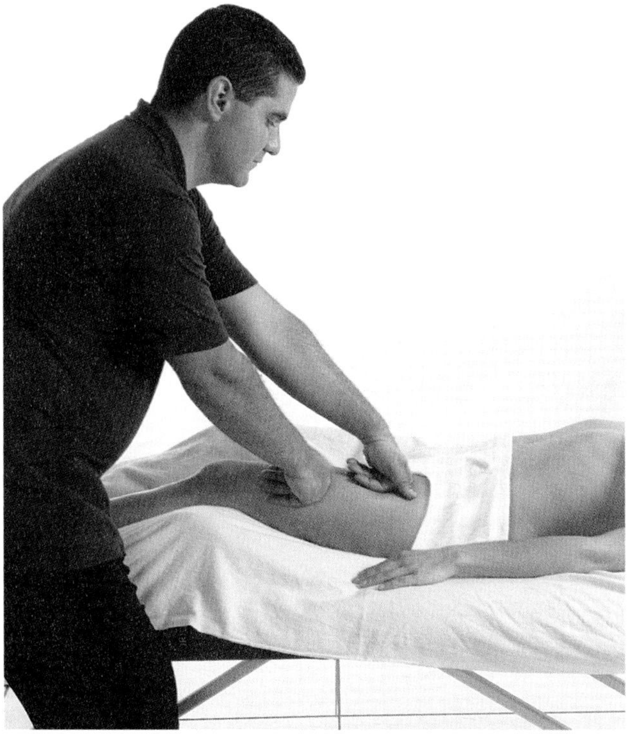

FIGURE 23-5 ■ Proceed with open-fist effleurage, moving up the thigh on the rectus femoris (wide view, to show body mechanics).

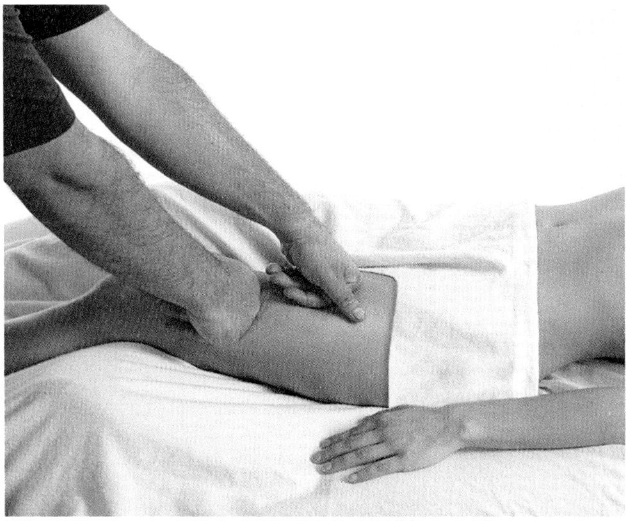

FIGURE 23-6 ■ Proceed with open-fist effleurage, moving up the thigh on the rectus femoris (close-up view, to show hand placement).

QUADRICEPS DYSFUNCTION ROUTINE

8 Perform deep-stripping up the thigh (Figure 23-7).

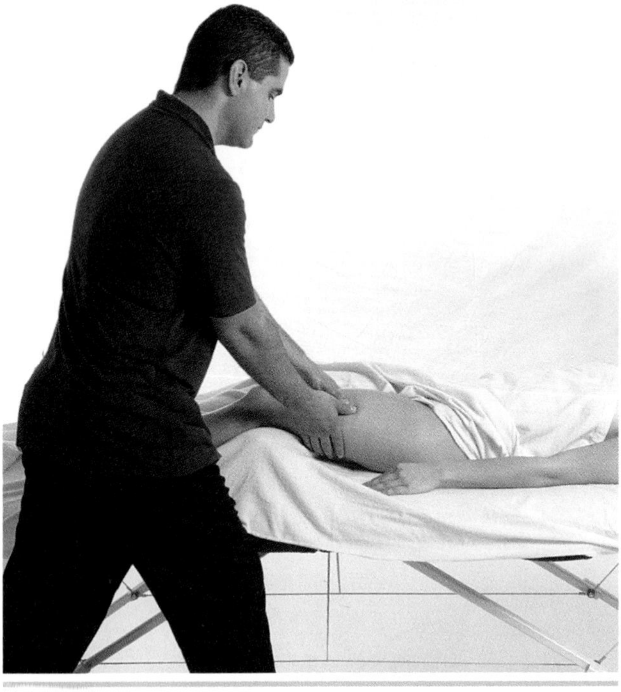

FIGURE 23-7 ■

QUADRICEPS DYSFUNCTION ROUTINE

9 Slightly move the rectus femoris to the side and perform circular friction to the vastus intermedius (under the rectus).
10 Effleurage and perform concluding strokes.
11 Stretch the quadriceps, hamstrings, and adductor groups.

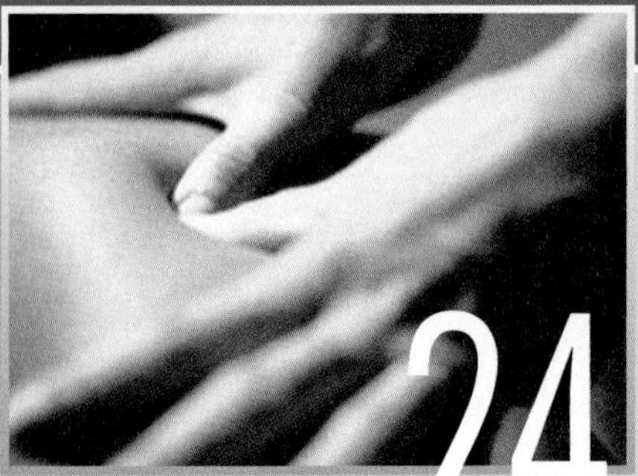

CHAPTER 24

ILIOTIBIAL BAND DISORDER

OUTLINE

Definition and symptoms
Indications
Contraindications
Iliotibial band disorder routine

KEY TERMS

Iliotibial band disorder
Peripheral vascular disease

OBJECTIVES

Upon completion of this chapter the reader will have the information necessary to:

1 **Define common iliotibial (IT) band disorder causes**
2 **Describe common IT band disorder symptoms**
3 **Identify common IT band disorder routine indications**
4 **Classify common IT band disorder routine contraindications**
5 **Understand and perform an IT band disorder routine**

DEFINITION AND SYMPTOMS

Iliotibial band disorder is an inflammatory condition that is the result of friction (rubbing) of the band of the iliotibial (IT) tendon over the outer bone (femur). Although the syndrome may be caused by direct injury to the knee, it is most often caused by the stress of long-term overuse (e.g., from sports training). Symptoms include an ache or burning sensation at the side of the knee during activity, pain radiating from the lateral hip down to the lateral aspect of the knee. A "snap" may also be felt when the knee is bent and then straightened. Methods of treatment include massage therapy, stretching, rest, or surgery.

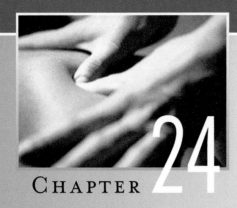

Indications

- Pain on the lateral aspect of the thigh
- Knee pain
- Muscle tightness
- Reduced knee and hip range of motion (ROM)

Contraindications

- Edema
- Open lesions
- Acute knee sprains
- Varicose veins
- Peripheral vascular disease (PVD)

ILIOTIBIAL BAND DISORDER ROUTINE

POSITION: CLIENT IS SIDE-LYING (SIDE BEING WORKED EXPOSED)

PROCEDURE:

1 Make sure client is comfortable by placing a pillow or bolster between knees for support.
2 Effleurage the entire side of the thigh from the knee to the iliac crest.
3 This area is usually very sensitive, so proceed with caution by thumb-stripping up the IT band from the knee to the tensor fascia latae (TFL) muscle (Figure 24-1).

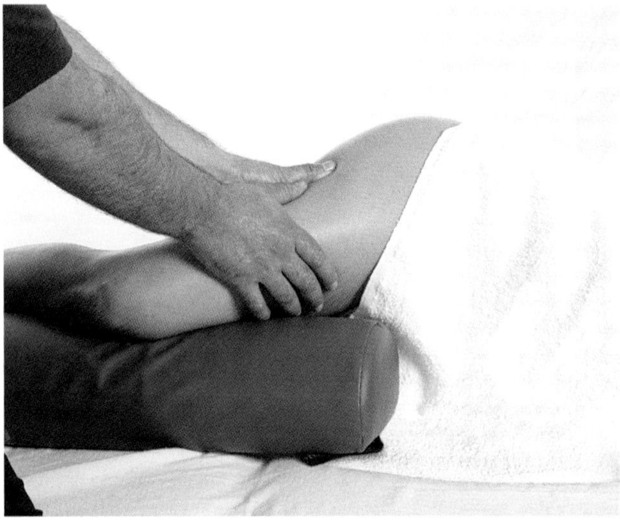

FIGURE 24-1 ■

4 Use cross-fiber friction on the entire band, starting on the lateral knee and concluding on the TFL muscle.
5 Displace the IT band and perform circular friction just underneath it (Figure 24-2).

ILIOTIBIAL BAND DISORDER ROUTINE

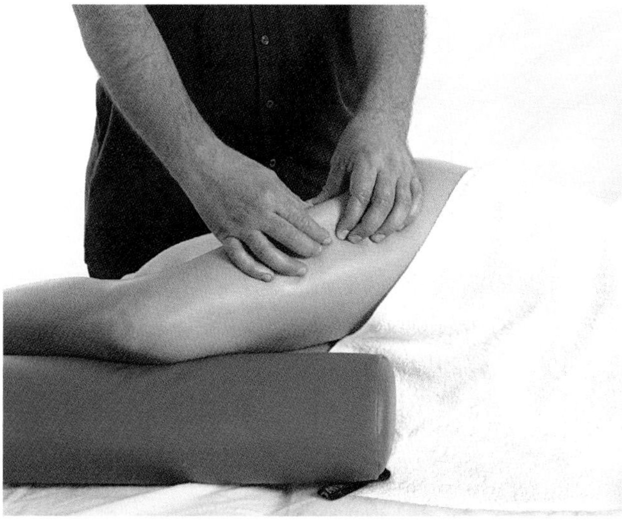

FIGURE 24-2 ■

6 Thumb-strip (with-fiber friction) the belly of the TFL muscle (Figure 24-3).

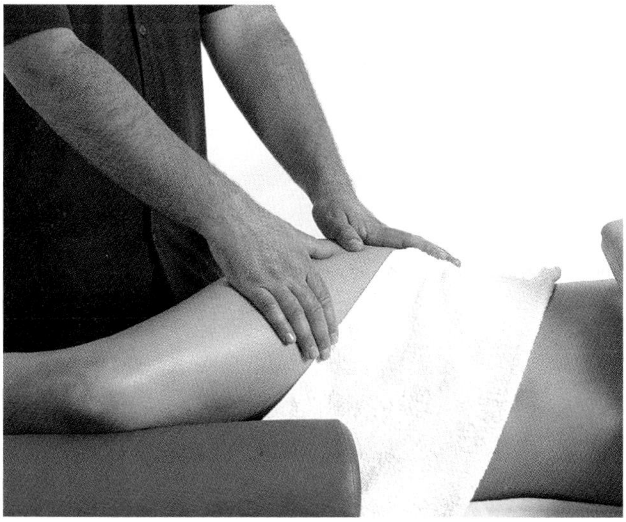

FIGURE 24-3 ■

7 Use cross-fiber friction on the origin of the TFL muscle.
8 Perform deep effleurage over the entire medial thigh.
9 Perform concluding strokes.
10 Stretch the TFL muscle and IT band.

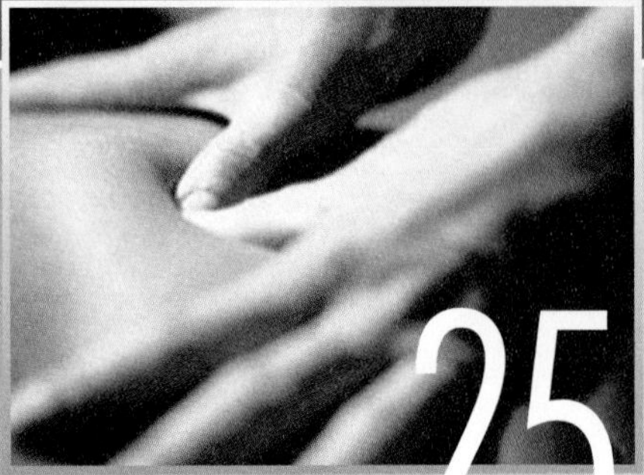

CHAPTER 25

PATELLOFEMORAL DYSFUNCTION

OUTLINE

Definition and symptoms
Indications
Contraindications
Patellofemoral dysfunction routine

KEY TERM

Patellofemoral dysfunction

OBJECTIVES

Upon completion of this chapter the reader will have the information necessary to:

1. **Define common patellofemoral dysfunction causes**
2. **Describe common patellofemoral dysfunction symptoms**
3. **Identify common patellofemoral dysfunction routine indications**
4. **Classify common patellofemoral dysfunction routine contraindications**
5. **Understand and perform a patellofemoral dysfunction routine**

DEFINITION AND SYMPTOMS

Patellofemoral dysfunction results from an injury that occurs at the articulation between the patella (kneecap) and the underlying femur. The patella is a diamond-shaped bone that lies in an identically shaped groove in front of the femur. The patella functions as a pulley to assist the quadriceps by providing a mechanical advantage for added strength. Patellofemoral dysfunction may occur when the patella is forced with excessive pressure against the underlying femur or when it rubs excessively on one side of the groove. This causes an irritation of the cartilage of the patella, resulting in inflammation and pain.

Excessive pressure of the patella against the femur could also result from excessively tight quadriceps muscles.

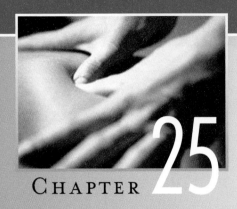

Indications

- Knee pain
- Reduced range of motion (ROM)
- Tight quads
- Frequent cramping
- Inability to "lock" the knee

Contraindications

- Acute edema
- Acute ligament strain
- Open lesions
- Varicose veins
- Peripheral vascular disease

PATELLOFEMORAL DYSFUNCTION ROUTINE

POSITION: CLIENT IS SUPINE

PROCEDURE:

1 Effleurage the quadriceps (hand-over-hand).
2 Perform open-fisting technique up the thigh.
3 Perform deep petrissage on the quadriceps.
4 Thumb-strip (with-fiber friction) vastus lateralis, rectus femoris, and vastus medialis at an angle (moving laterally) (Figure 25-1).

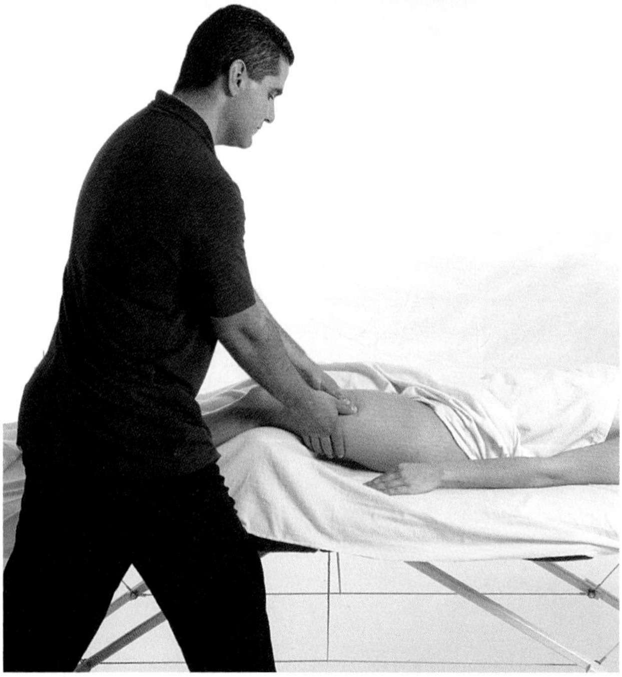

FIGURE 25-1

PATELLOFEMORAL DYSFUNCTION ROUTINE

5 Find and deactivate all active trigger points in the quadriceps group (Figure 25-2).

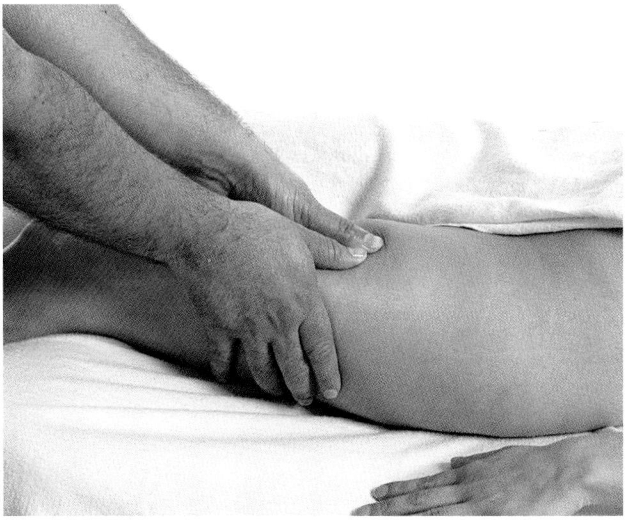

FIGURE 25-2

6 Place knee in flexion and use cross-fiber friction over the rectus femoris origin.
7 Remove bolster under the knee being worked and position the leg back down on the table.
8 Displace the patella medial to lateral "only" and use circular friction under patella (knee should be on a flat surface). Repeat 2 to 3 times (Figure 25-3).

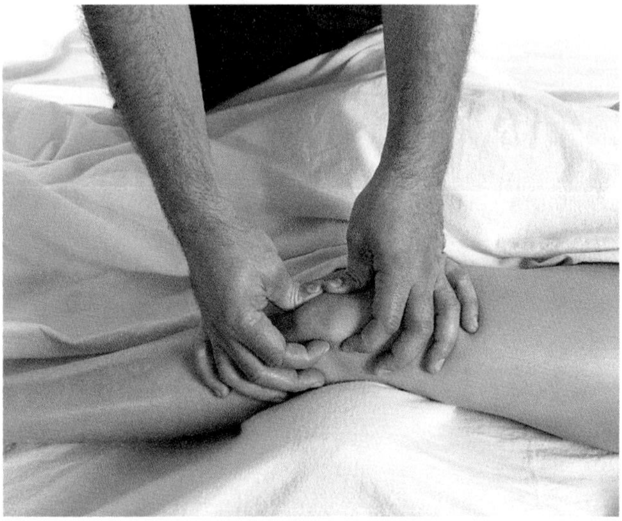

FIGURE 25-3 ■

POSITION: CLIENT IS NOW PRONE

PROCEDURE:

1 Apply effleurage to the hamstrings, inferior to superior.
2 Perform petrissage and deep open-fisting on the hamstrings.
3 Find the belly of the three hamstrings and thumb-strip from inferior to superior (popliteal toward ischium) the entire area.
4 Find and deactivate all active trigger points in the hamstring muscles.
5 Place hand over leg and ask client to resist in order to find the origin of hamstring; once found use cross-fiber friction on hamstring origin (ischial tuberosity), making sure not to use cross-fiber friction on bone (repeat for insertion).
6 Effleurage and perform concluding strokes on the area worked (Figures 25-4 and 25-5).

PATELLOFEMORAL DYSFUNCTION ROUTINE

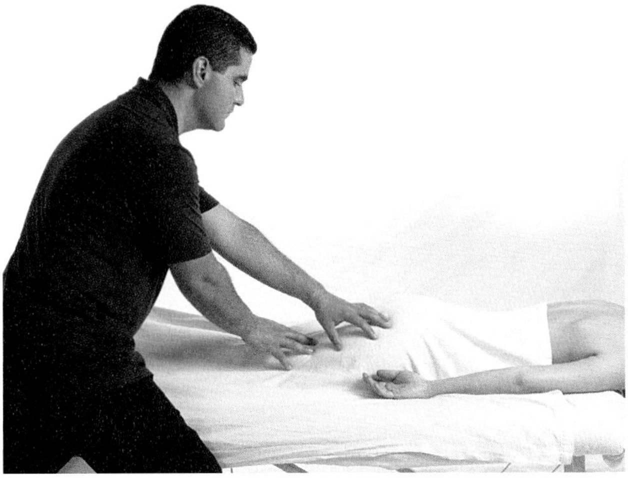

FIGURE 25-4 ■ Effleurage and perform concluding strokes on the area worked.

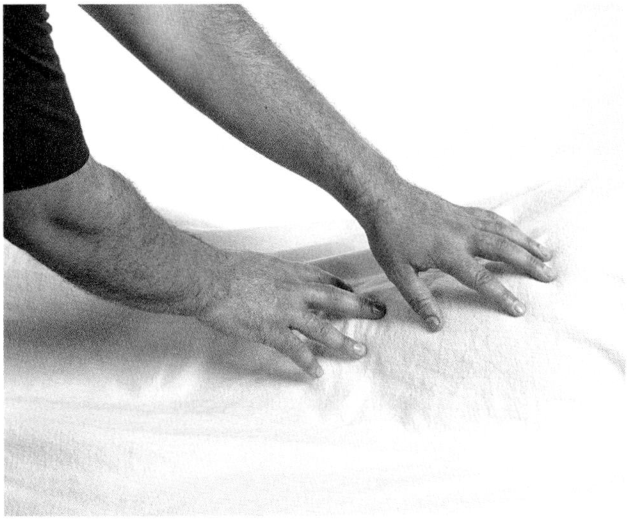

FIGURE 25-5 ■ Effleurage and perform concluding strokes on the area worked.

7 Conclude treatment by stretching the hamstrings, quadriceps, iliotibial band, and adductor groups.

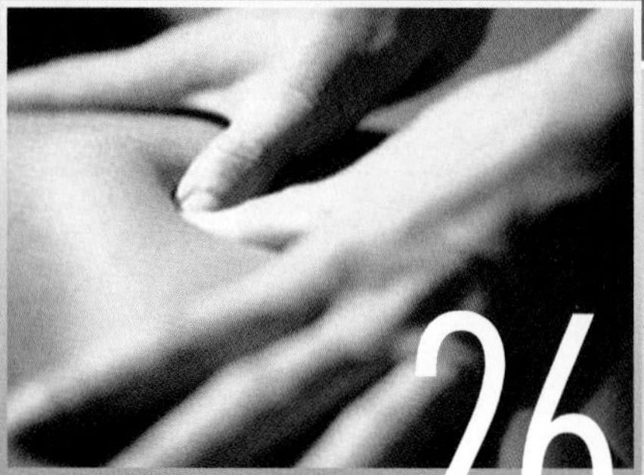

CHAPTER 26

SHIN SPLINTS

OUTLINE

Definition and symptoms
Indications
Contraindications
Shin splints routine

KEY TERMS

Shin splints
PNF

OBJECTIVES

Upon completion of this chapter the reader will have the information necessary to:

1. **Define common shin splints causes**
2. **Describe common shin splints symptoms**
3. **Identify common shin splints routine indications**
4. **Classify common shin splints routine contraindications**
5. **Understand and perform a shin splints routine**

DEFINITION AND SYMPTOMS

Shin splints (medial tibial stress syndrome) are an inflammation of the thin layer of tissue that covers the bone (periosteum). A shin splint is an injury or strain that occurs along or just behind the inner (medial) edge of the shin (tibia). The pain usually spans about 3 to 4 inches. Shin splints result from exercise and overuse of the involved leg(s). Studies show that shin splints commonly affect runners, aerobic dancers, and athletes or people who heavily utilize their legs when exercising.

Certain factors contribute to the onset of shin splints, including excessive exercising, dancing, overuse (fatiguing the muscle), an extremely flat foot or abnormally rigid arch, knock knees, or bow legs in runners, aerobic dancers, or military personnel (due to extraneous exercising and poor stretching). Treatments include massage, stretching, or taking anti-inflammatory medications.

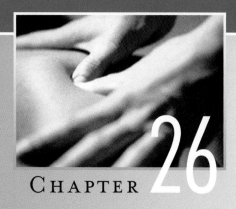

Indications

- Strains
- Knee pain
- Tightness
- Loss of range of motion (ROM)

Contraindications

- Edema
- Sprains
- Varicose veins
- Acute injury

SHIN SPLINTS ROUTINE

POSITION: CLIENT IS SUPINE

PROCEDURE:

1 Use slow myofascial release (MFR) inferiorly to superiorly over the entire anterior leg area (twice on each side of the leg) (Figure 26-1).

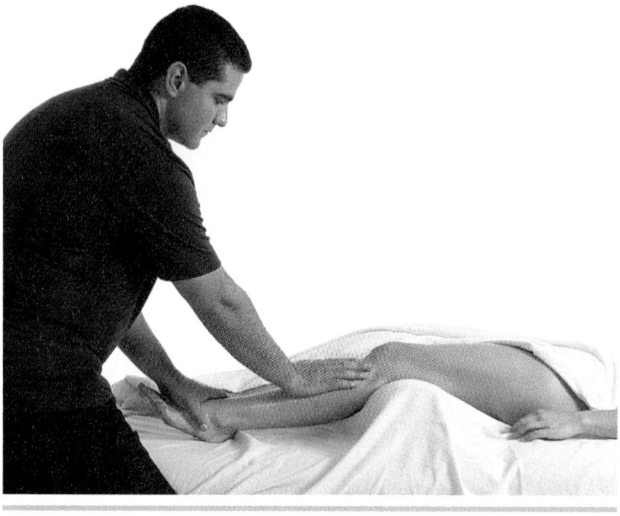

FIGURE 26-1

NOTE: Myofascial release should be performed with a minimum amount of cream or 100% cocoa butter.

2 Use slow MFR medially to laterally one side at a time (once only).

3 Skin-roll the entire area if the client tolerates it (Figure 26-2).

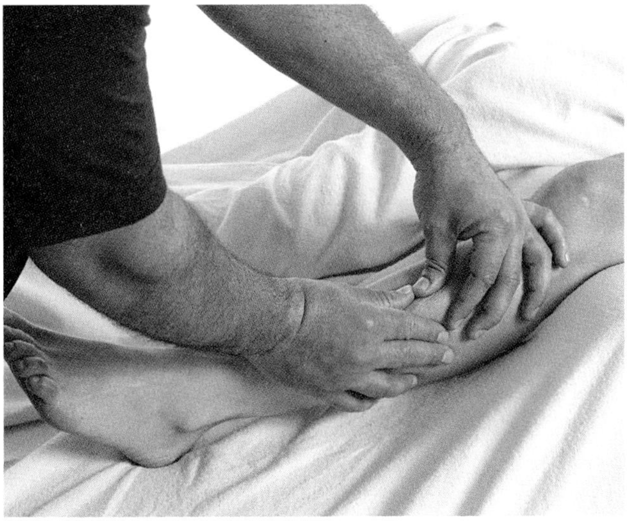

FIGURE 26-2 ■

4 Effleurage the entire tibialis anterior area.
5 Perform muscle-sculpting (using deep effleurage) with palm upwards from the lateral malleolus to the head of the fibula.
6 Deep-strip the area between the tibialis anterior and extensor digitorum longus (lateral leg only) (Figure 26-3).

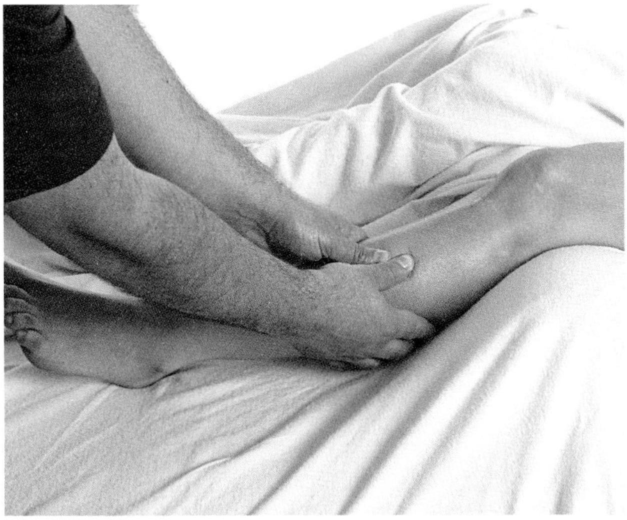

FIGURE 26-3 ■

SHIN SPLINTS ROUTINE

7 Apply parallel cross-fiber friction to the tendon insertions of the tibialis anterior, extensor hallucis longus, extensor digitorum longus, and peroneus tertius (Figure 26-4).

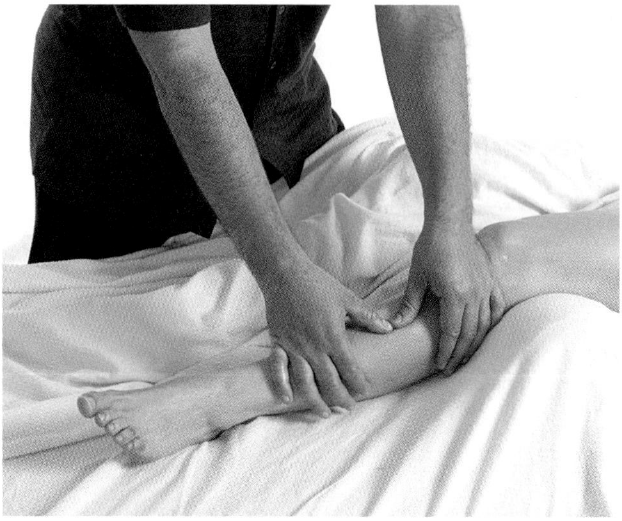

FIGURE 26-4

8 Find and deactivate all active trigger points along the tibialis anterior (lateral only) (Figure 26-5).

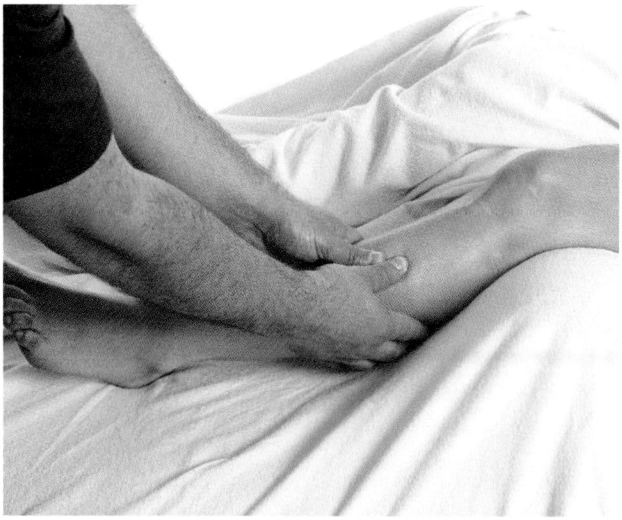

FIGURE 26-5

9 Effleurage the leg.

POSITION: CLIENT IS NOW SIDE-LYING

PROCEDURE:

1. With a bolster under the leg being worked, stand in front of the leg and place thumbs just above the tibial ridge (groove between the tibialis anterior and tibia).
2. Hook on the groove with thumbs and push from medial to lateral area about an inch until you feel it flip. Perform this technique on the entire groove.
3. Effleurage and perform concluding strokes.
4. Perform proprioceptive neuromuscular facilitation stretching to the tibialis anterior.

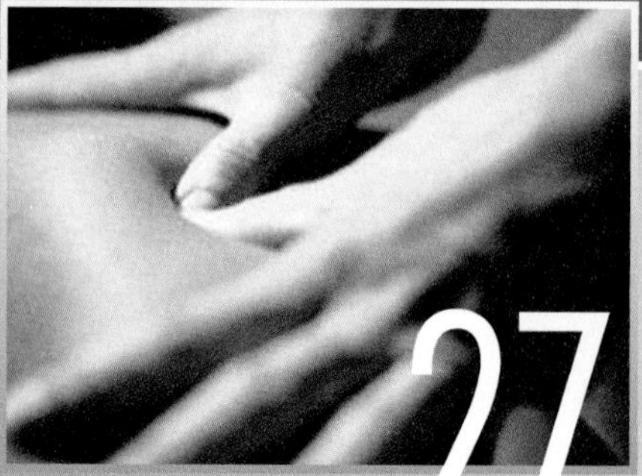

CHAPTER 27

PLANTAR FASCIITIS

OUTLINE

Definition and symptoms
Indications
Contraindications
Plantar fasciitis routine

KEY TERMS

Plantar fasciitis
Peripheral vascular disease

OBJECTIVES

Upon completion of this chapter the reader will have the information necessary to:

1. **Define common plantar fasciitis causes**
2. **Describe common plantar fasciitis symptoms**
3. **Identify common plantar fasciitis routine indications**
4. **Classify common plantar fasciitis routine contraindications**
5. **Understand and perform a plantar fasciitis routine**

DEFINITION AND SYMPTOMS

Plantar fasciitis is an inflammation of the plantar fascia, a thin layer of tough tissue supporting the arch of the foot. Repeated microscopic tears of the plantar fascia cause discomfort, pain, and scar tissue. This disorder is also referred to as "heel spurs"; however, this is not always accurate because bony growths on the heel may or may not be a factor.

The pain associated with plantar fasciitis is more noticeable at the beginning of an activity and lessens as the body warms up. Prolonged standing may cause heel pain as well. In more severe cases, the pain may worsen toward the end of the day.

There are a number of possible causes for plantar fasciitis, including tightness of the foot and calf,

Icon represents an area where extreme caution should be used to avoid damage or compression to underlying or neighboring vessels.

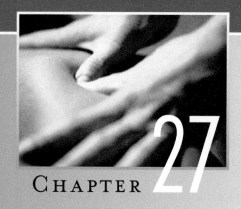

improper athletic training, stress on the arch, weakness of the foot, or injury. People with low arches, flat feet, or high arches are at increased risk of developing plantar fasciitis.

Indication

- Tight bands in the calf muscles
- Sub-acute injury
- Chronic injury
- Pain on the arch of the foot

Contraindications

- Varicose veins
- **Peripheral vascular disease (PVD)**
- History of blood clots
- Pregnancy
- Acute injuries

PLANTAR FASCIITIS ROUTINE

POSITION: CLIENT IS PRONE

PROCEDURE:

1. Effleurage the posterior leg muscles (hand-over-hand).
2. Petrissage the gastrocnemius muscle.
3. Perform deep-stripping to the Achilles tendon and gastrocnemius, making sure to stay away from the popliteal area and the midline of the gastrocnemius (Figure 27-1).

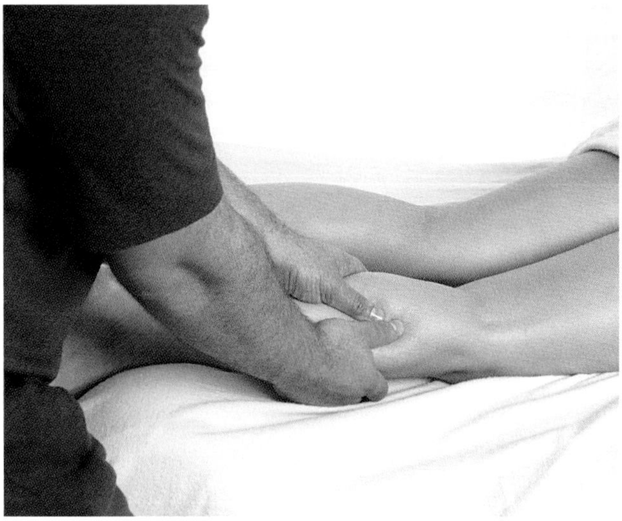

FIGURE 27-1

PLANTAR FASCIITIS ROUTINE

4 Find and deactivate all active trigger points in the gastrocnemius, soleus, and plantaris muscles.
5 Being cautious with the popliteal area, pincer-grip and friction the head of the gastrocnemius twice on each side (lateral and then medial) (Figure 27-2).

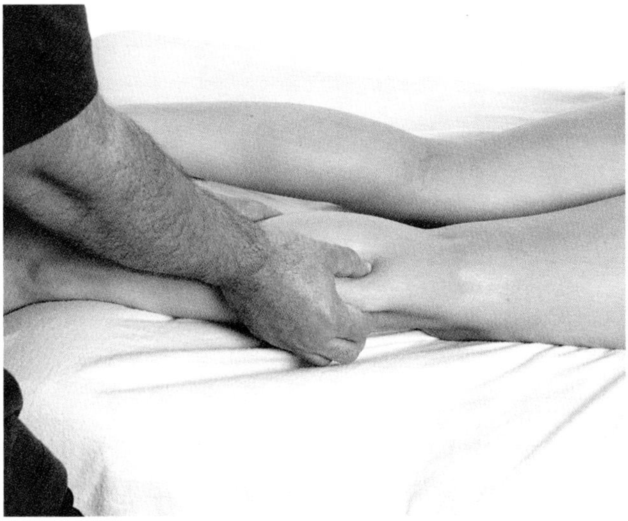

FIGURE 27-2

PLANTAR FASCIITIS ROUTINE

6 Effleurage the entire muscle.
7 Warm up the plantar surface of the foot with effleurage and digital-stripping (Figure 27-3).

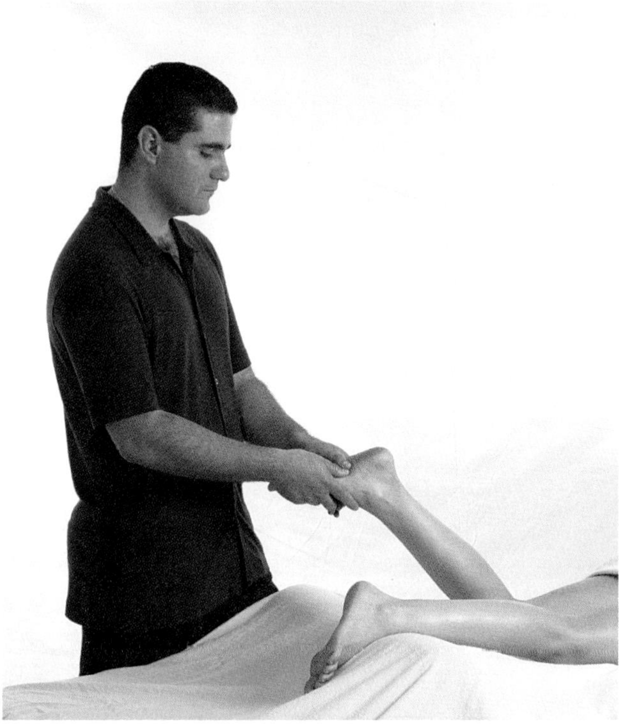

FIGURE 27-3 ■

8 Scoop with thumb (may use T-bar) superiorly to inferiorly on plantar surface, starting on calcaneus and stopping at metatarsals (Figure 27-4).

Be careful with medial surface; it may be extremely sensitive.

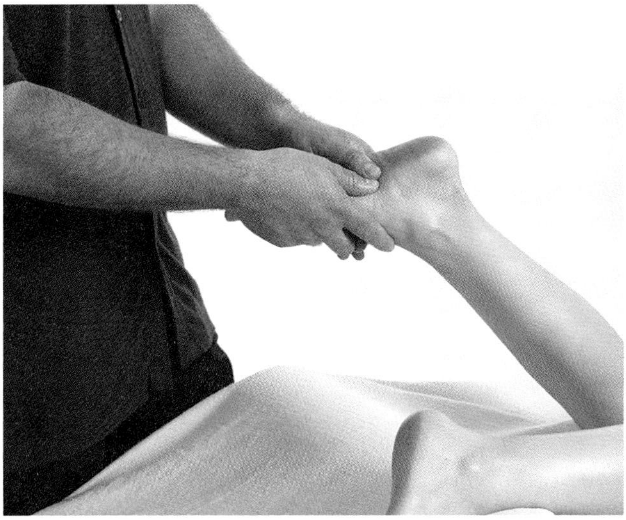

FIGURE 27-4

9 Effleurage and stretch toes in dorsiflexion direction for fascia release.

10 Conclude by stretching the gastrocnemius and plantar section of the foot.

CHAPTER 28

FIBROMYALGIA SYNDROME

OUTLINE

Definition and symptoms
Indications
Contraindications
Fibromyalgia syndrome routine

KEY TERMS

Fibromyalgia syndrome
Hoku point

OBJECTIVES

Upon completion of this chapter the reader will have the information necessary to:

1. **Define common fibromyalgia syndrome causes**
2. **Describe common fibromyalgia syndrome symptoms**
3. **Identify common fibromyalgia syndrome routine indications**
4. **Classify common fibromyalgia syndrome routine contraindications**
5. **Understand and perform a fibromyalgia syndrome routine**

DEFINITION AND SYMPTOMS

F**ibromyalgia** is a condition characterized by extensive pain in joints, muscles, tendons, dermatomes, and other soft tissues. Symptoms linked with **fibromyalgia syndrome** (FMS) include fatigue, morning stiffness, sleep problems, headaches, lack of motivation, numbness in hands and feet, depression, and anxiety. The most common are disabling fatigue, persistent muscle and joint pain, and severe problems of forgetfulness, irritability, and depression. This condition is more common in women than in men and generally occurs between the ages of 35 and 60; however, there have been cases where FMS has started in the teenage years. Treatments include low-dose drugs, exercise, visualization, massage therapy, counseling, stress management, and support groups.

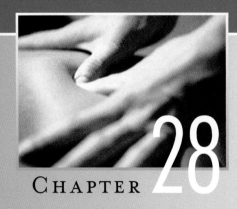

Considerations for massage:

- Tender points can be very sensitive; therefore, make sure to be in constant communication with the patient throughout the treatment.
- People with FMS tire easily. Be sensitive to fatigue level and stop the treatment if paint tolerance level is reached.
- Techniques involved should be long, slow strokes.
- The environment should be quiet.
- There are approximately 18 to 20 tender points in the body that can be directly linked to FMS. Hold these points for 30 to 60 seconds unless the client asks you otherwise.

Indications

- Fatigue
- Muscle tenderness
- Active related tender points
- Headaches
- Anxiety

Contraindications

- Viral-like illness
- History of cancer
- Open lesions

POSITION: CLIENT IS SUPINE (15 MINUTES)

PROCEDURE:

NOTE: Client may be dressed for this routine.

1 Traction the neck with an occipital stretch. Make sure to contact the tender spot on either side of the head along the occipital ridge (Figures 28-1 and 28-2).

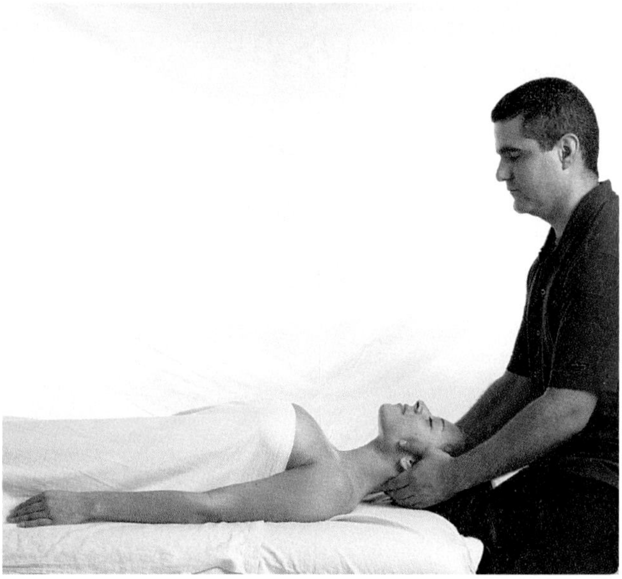

FIGURE 28-1 ■ Proper body mechanics when starting the fibromyalgia syndrome routine.

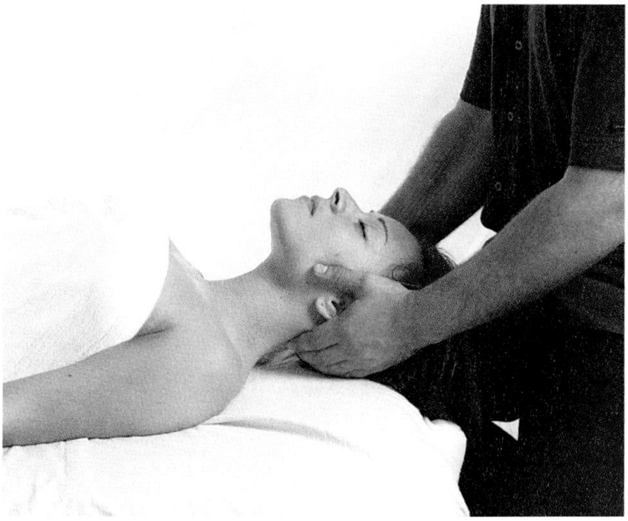

FIGURE 28-2 ■ Contact the tender spot on either side of the head along the occipital ridge.

2 Stretch the neck chin to chest (Figure 28-3).

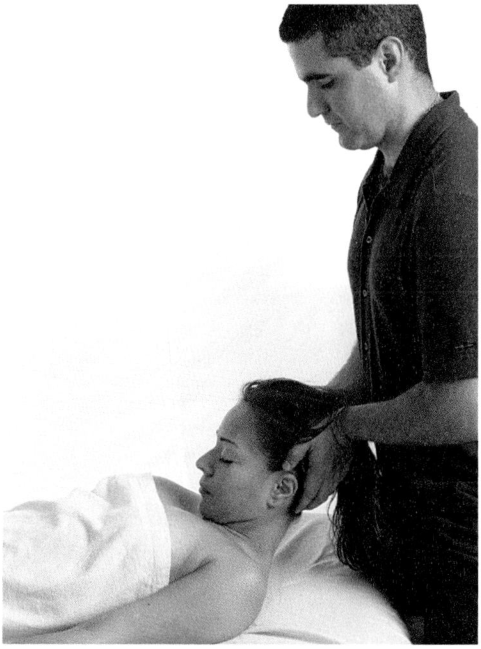

FIGURE 28-3 ■

3 Stretch the neck laterally at an angle (do not force it) (Figure 28-4).

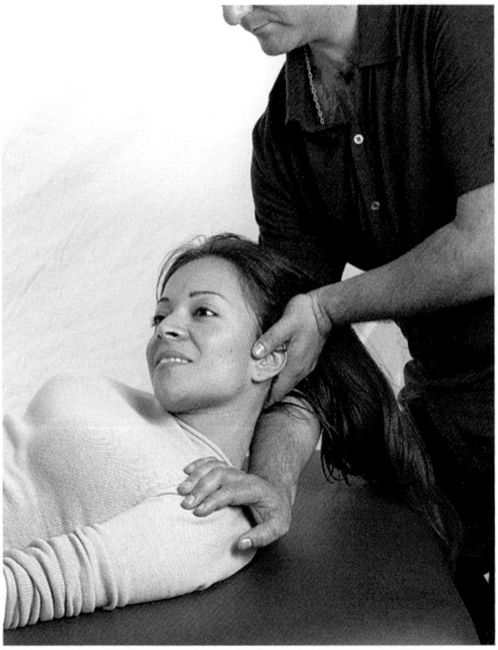

FIGURE 28-4

FIBROMYALGIA SYNDROME ROUTINE

4 Perform lateral stroking of the forehead.
5 Apply slow circular friction to the masseter and temporalis area. Accompany with a temporal mandibular joint and masseter stretch.
6 Place pressure to the tender spot at the top of the sternocleidomastoid muscle posterior to the mandible.
7 Depress shoulders evenly with the flat of the hands. Hold for 30 seconds and follow with a gentle rocking movement (Figure 28-5).

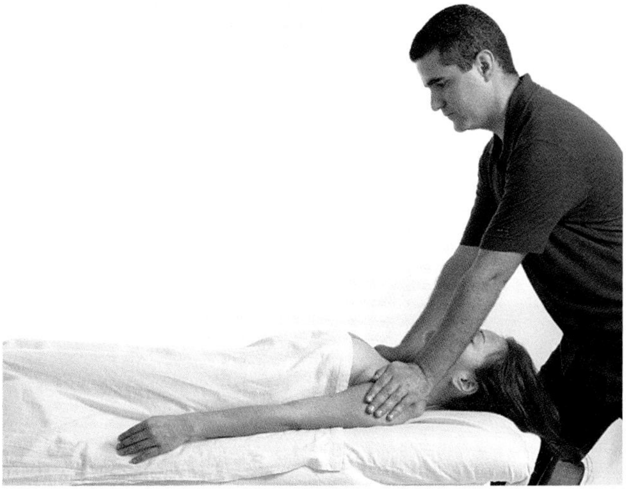

FIGURE 28-5

FIBROMYALGIA SYNDROME ROUTINE

8 Compress tender point located at the mid-shoulders (upper trapezius).
9 Hold tender point at the lower portion of the SCM muscle (sternoclavicular region).
10 Traction the arm and follow with range of motion from inferior to superior to lateral (no adduction).
11 Hold tender point at the lateral epicondyle of the humerus.
12 Gently massage the hand with the intent to relax the whole being (Figure 28-6).

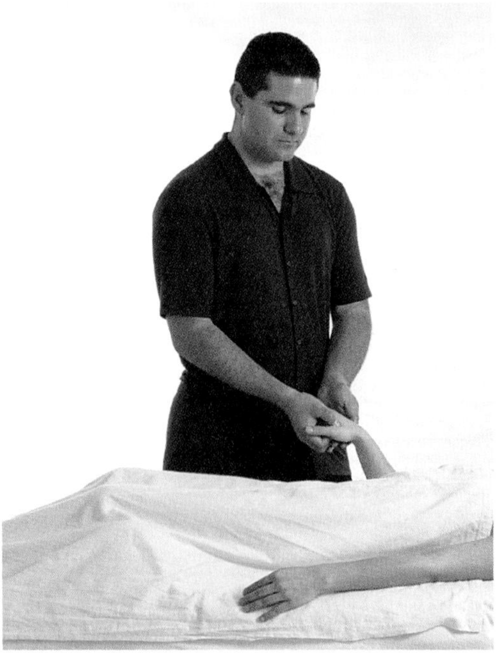

FIGURE 28-6

13 Hold **Hoku point** at the crevice of the thumb (Figure 28-7). This is located on the highest elevated point of the hump produced by adducting the thumb.

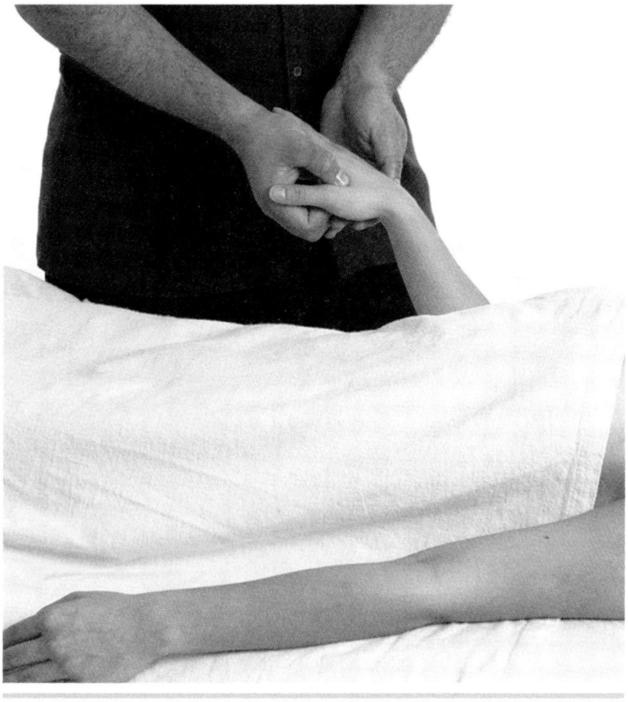

FIGURE 28-7

14 Apply slow nerve strokes from above the shoulders to beyond the hand.
15 Place hand gently on the solar plexus (diaphragm) and gently rock (other hand may be placed on the forehead if desired) (Figures 28-8 and 28-9).

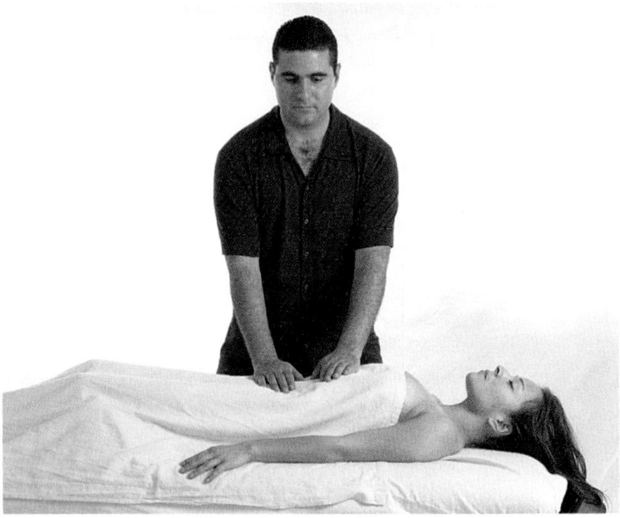

FIGURE 28-8 ■ Place hand gently on the solar plexus (diaphragm).

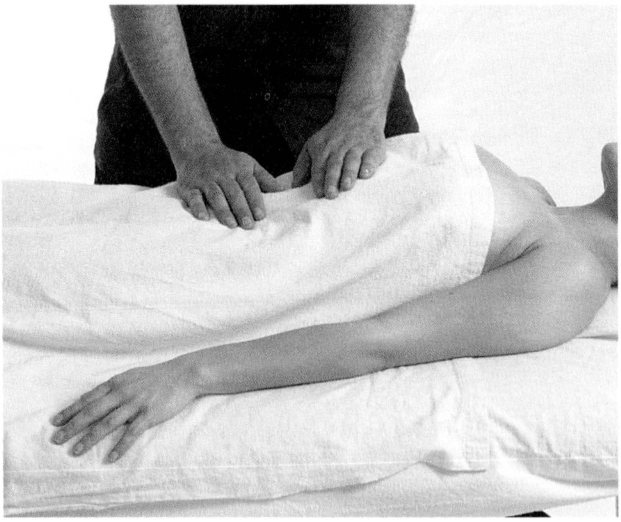

FIGURE 28-9 ■ Gently rock.

16 Traction both legs together; use straight traction as well as lateral.

17 Gently and slowly massage the feet following the metatarsal spaces. Do not use any digging, high pressure, or deep friction.

POSITION: CLIENT IS NOW PRONE (15 MINUTES)

PROCEDURE:

1 Perform Achilles tendon stretch (Figure 28-10).

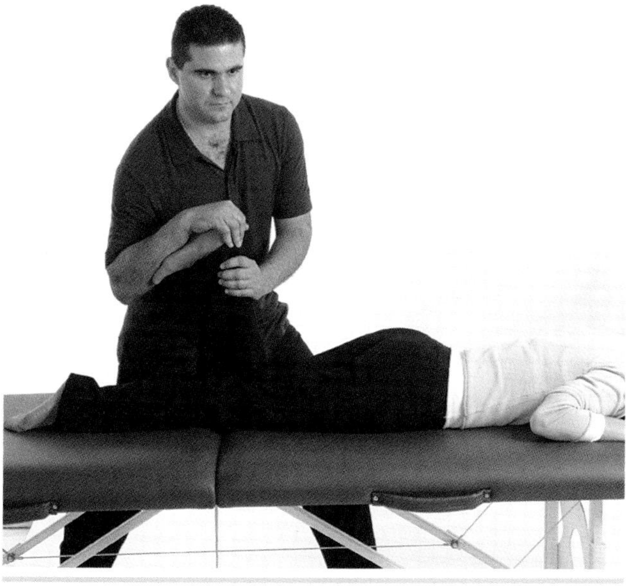

FIGURE 28-10

2 Perform knee shake with the knee bent at a 90-degree angle (Figure 28-11).

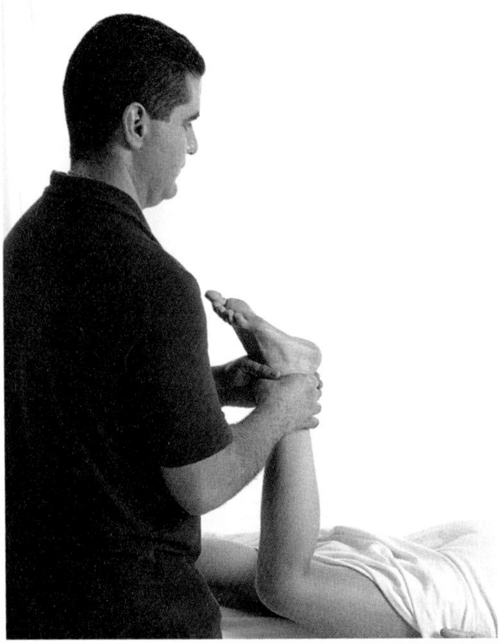

FIGURE 28-11

3 Hold the tender spot at the sciatic notch followed by the ones on the greater trochanter located on the anterior part of the femur.
4 Perform slow nerve strokes from above the buttocks to beyond the feet (Figures 28-12 and 28-13).

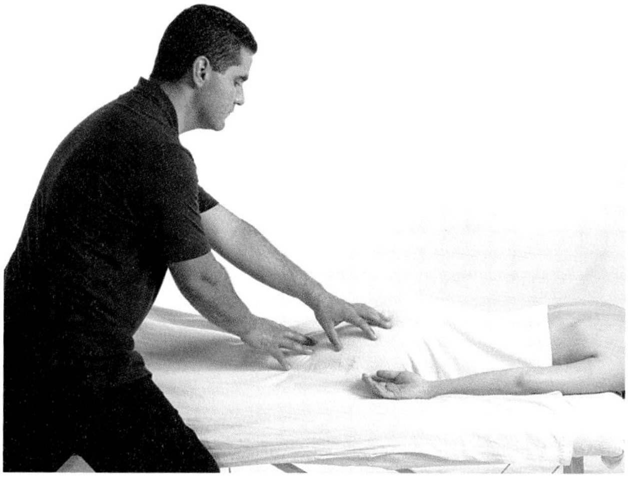

FIGURE 28-12 ■ Proper body position when performing slow nerve strokes.

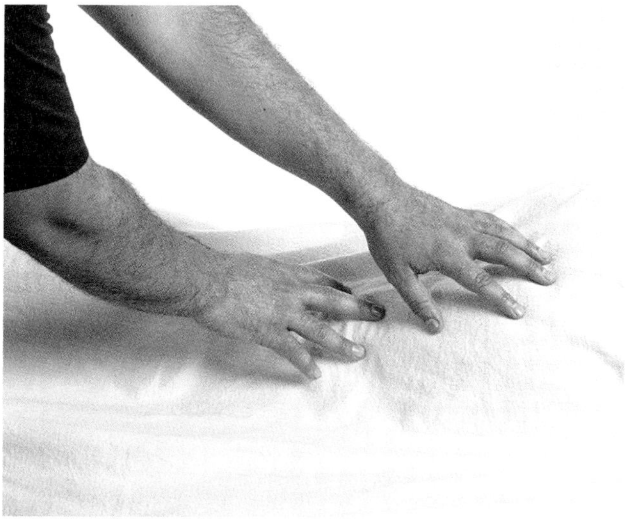

FIGURE 28-13 ■ Proper hand position when performing slow nerve strokes.

5 Perform lumbar stretch with the flats of the palms (4 times) (Figure 28-14).

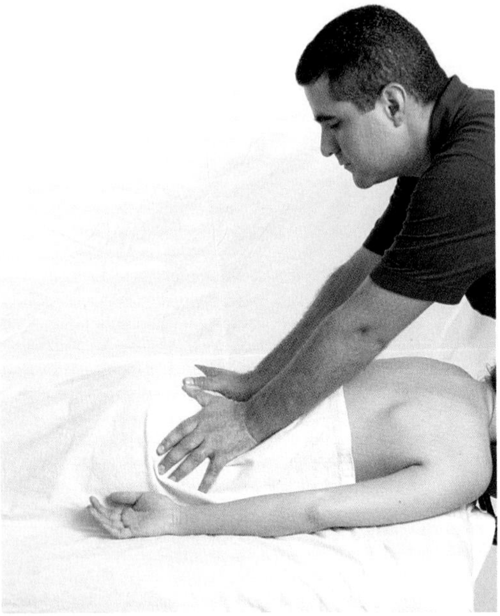

FIGURE 28-14 ■

6 Perform a gentle trapezius squeeze (Figures 28-15 and 28-16).

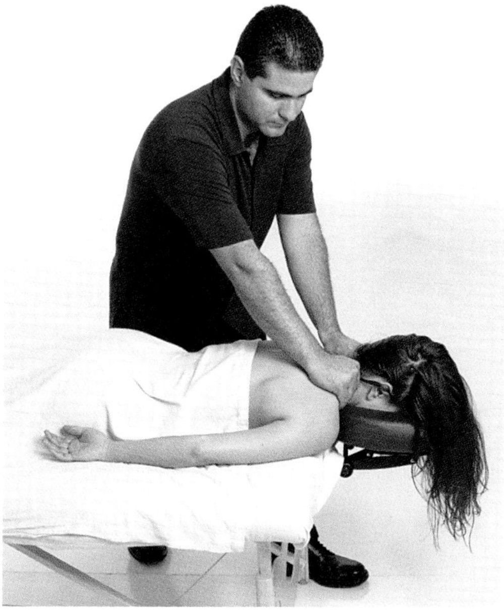

FIGURE 28-15 ■ Position of client and practitioner for trapezius squeeze.

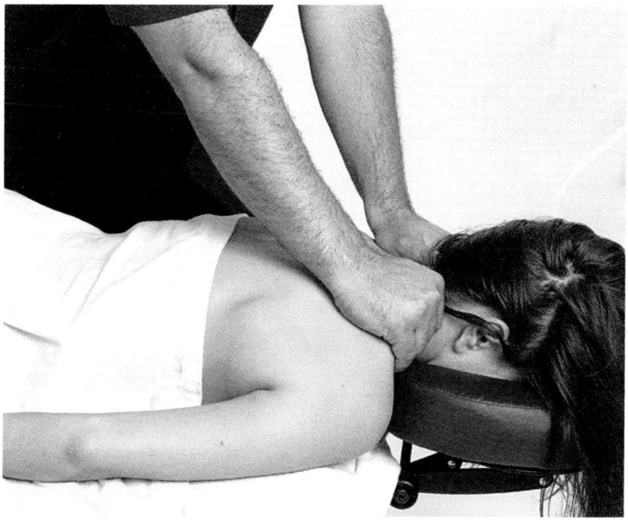

FIGURE 28-16 ■ Hand position for trapezius squeeze.

FIBROMYALGIA SYNDROME ROUTINE

7 Compress tender point in the rhomboid area near the mid-vertebral border of the scapula.
8 Apply with-fiber friction alongside the spine with the ulnar edge of the hand superiorly to inferiorly (Figures 28-17 and 28-18).

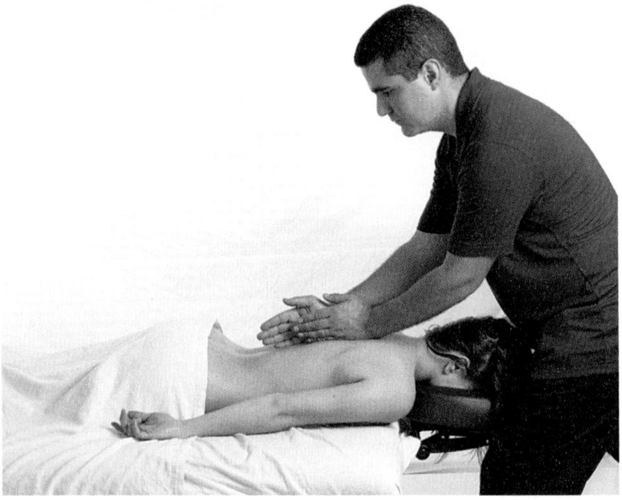

FIGURE 28-17 ■ Proper body position for performing friction alongside the spine.

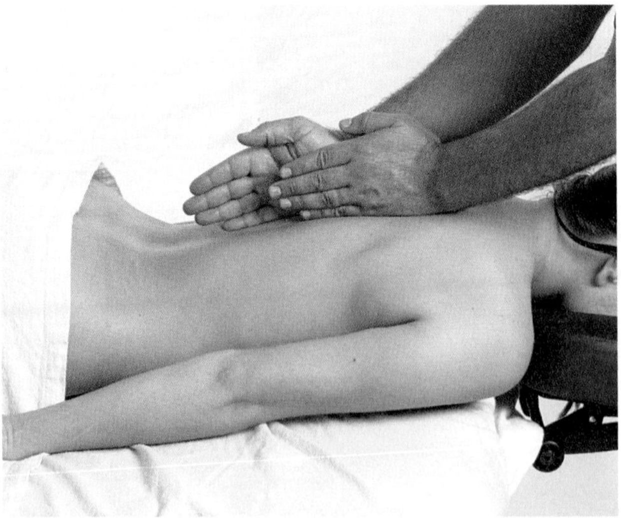

FIGURE 28-18 ■ Proper hand position for performing friction alongside the spine.

FIBROMYALGIA SYNDROME ROUTINE

9 Compress the tender point at the highest point of the iliac crest.
10 Perform a posterior neck squeeze and stretch.
11 Perform sacral traction (Figures 28-19 and 28-20).

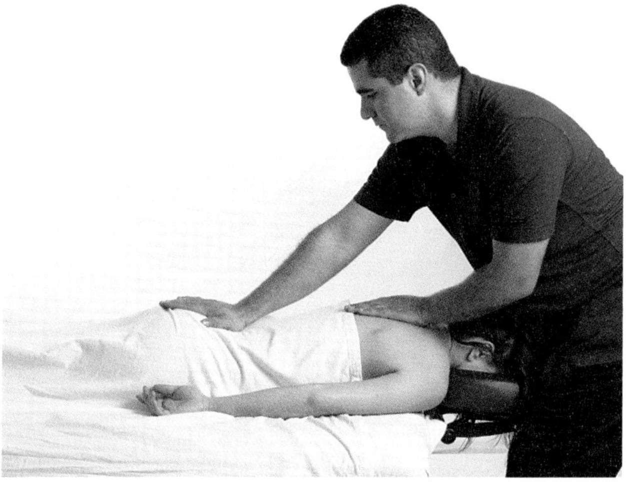

FIGURE 28-19 ■ Proper body and hand position for performing sacral traction.

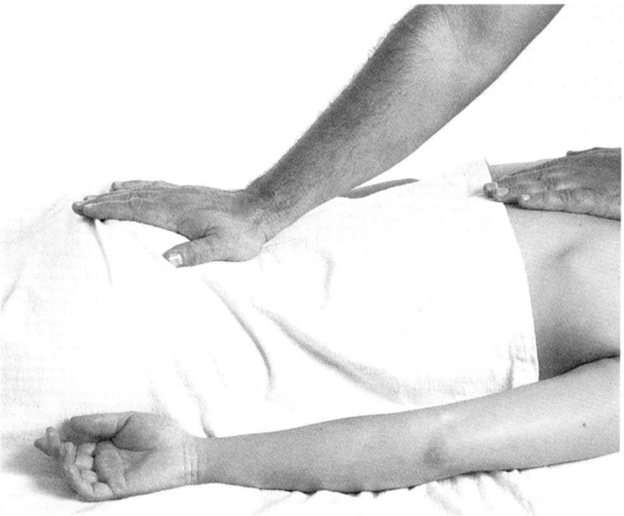

FIGURE 28-20 ■ Performing sacral traction.

FIBROMYALGIA SYNDROME ROUTINE

12 Apply long, slow nerve strokes from the shoulders down the entire posterior surface of the body all the way to the toes (2 times per side) (Figure 28-21).

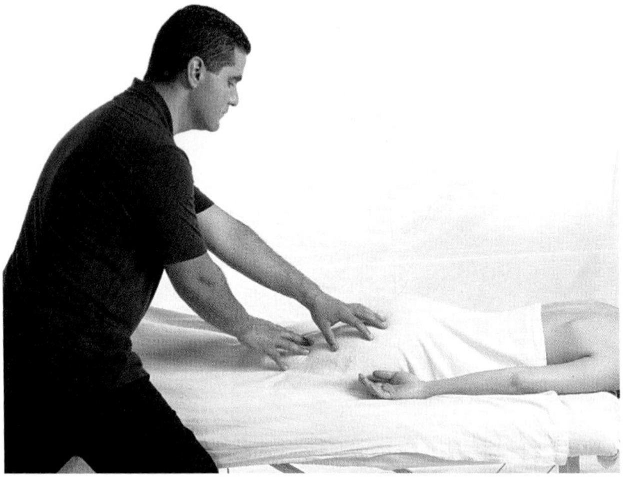

FIGURE 28-21

13 Place one hand over the lumbar region and the other over the thoracic and gently rock the body, then hold still for approximately one minute.

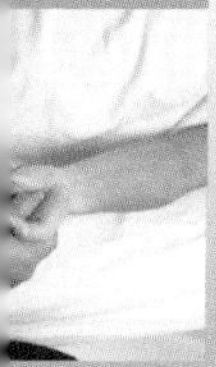
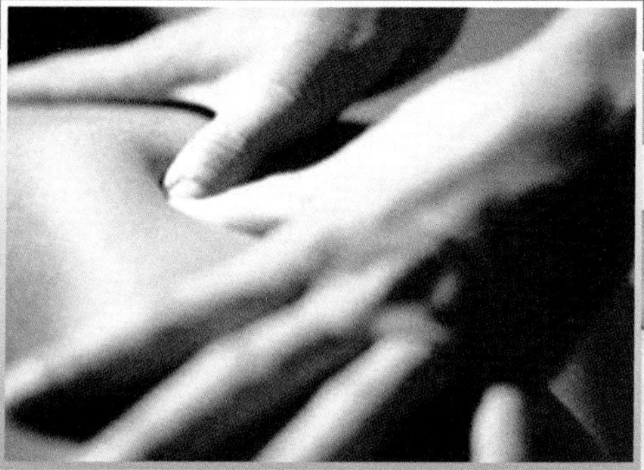
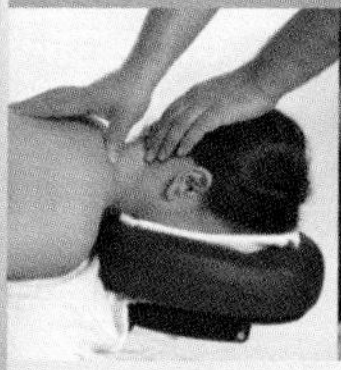
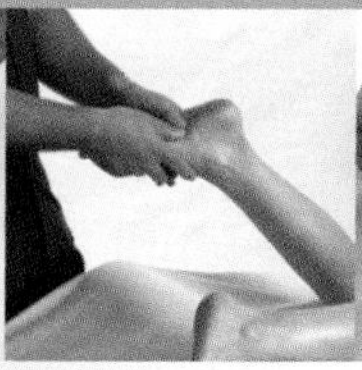
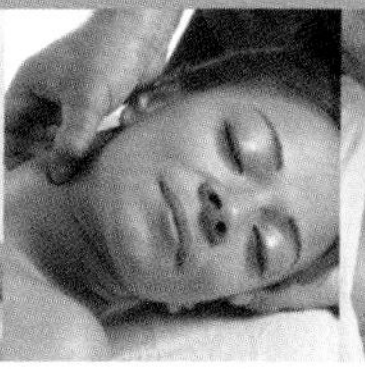
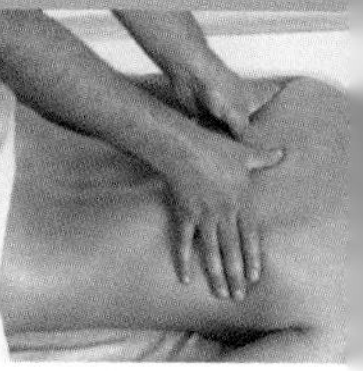

Part Three
STRETCHING

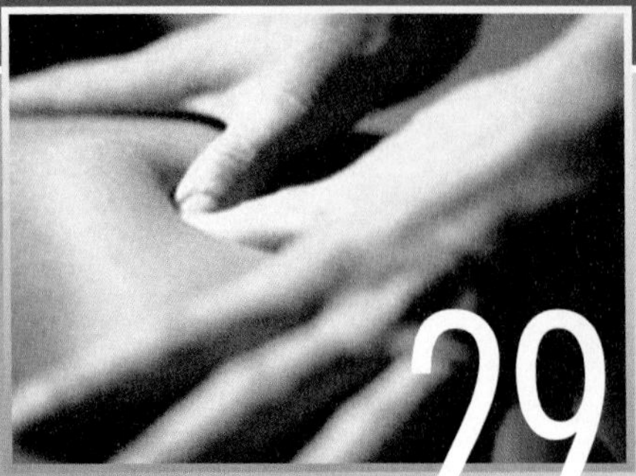

CHAPTER 29

STRETCHING

OUTLINE

Pectoralis
Hamstrings
Piriformis
Rotator cuff
Iliopsoas
Quadriceps
Cervical
Lateral cervical
Gastrocnemius
Back
Extensors of the hand
Flexors of the hand
Lower back
Sacral and lower back
Side-lying spinal stretch

KEY TERMS

Proprioceptive neuromuscular facilitation
Ballistic
Spinal torquing

OBJECTIVES

Upon completion of this chapter the reader will have the information necessary to:

1. **Define common stretching techniques**
2. **Describe common "lack of stretching" symptoms**
3. **Identify common stretching indications**
4. **Classify common stretching contraindications**
5. **Understand and perform common stretching exercises**

DEFINITION AND SYMPTOMS

There are a variety of stretching styles and techniques intended to lengthen the fibers of the muscles to increase flexibility, blood flow, range of motion (ROM), and reduce the risk of injury. Stretches indicated here include developmental, static, **proprioceptive neuromuscular facilitation** (PNF), and easy; contraindicated stretches include lunges, **ballistic** (bouncing), and **spinal torquing.**

Stretching is often done in an effort to reduce the probability of injury, but if done incorrectly, it actually increases the chances of injury. Muscle should be warmed up for at least two to three minutes (walking or exercising) before stretching. This increases the blood flow to the area, making it easier for the muscles to stretch. Stretching must be performed before *and* after exercise; this helps reduce lactic acid buildup, increases healing time, and helps maintain good ROM.

When stretching is incorporated into a massage treatment, it must be performed after the massage session because the muscles are already warmed up and oxygenated and will respond better to being lengthened.

Not all stretches are beneficial, however. Ballistic stretching (bouncing) causes micro-tears in the muscle fiber and which develop into scar tissue, which then reduces ROM in the joint.

The following stretches can be used to increase the treatment effect of massage.

PECTORALIS (Figures 29-1 and 29-2)

Can be performed with the following routines:

- Thoracic outlet syndrome
- Frozen shoulder

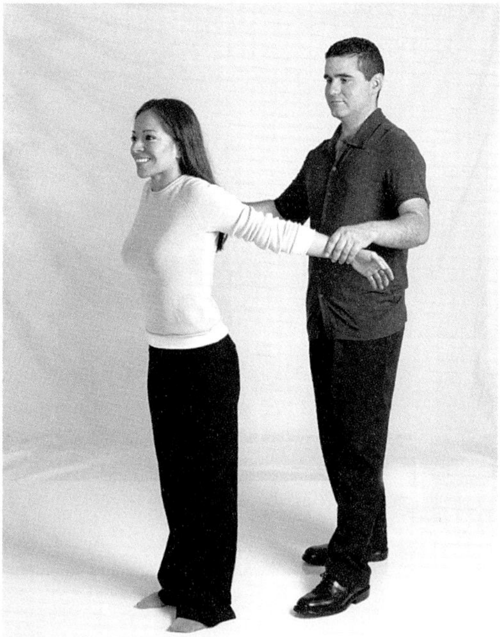

FIGURE 29-1

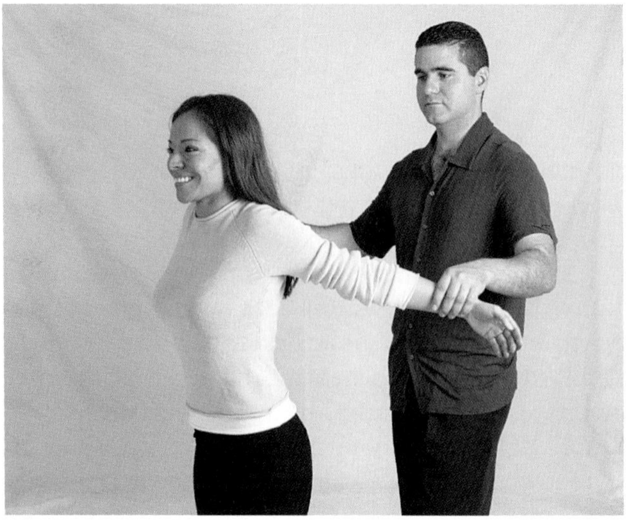

FIGURE 29-2 ■

- Rotator cuff tear
- Kyphosis
- Scoliosis

HAMSTRINGS (Figures 29-3 and 29-4)

Can be performed with the following routines:

- Lordosis
- Lower back pain
- Iliopsoas disorder

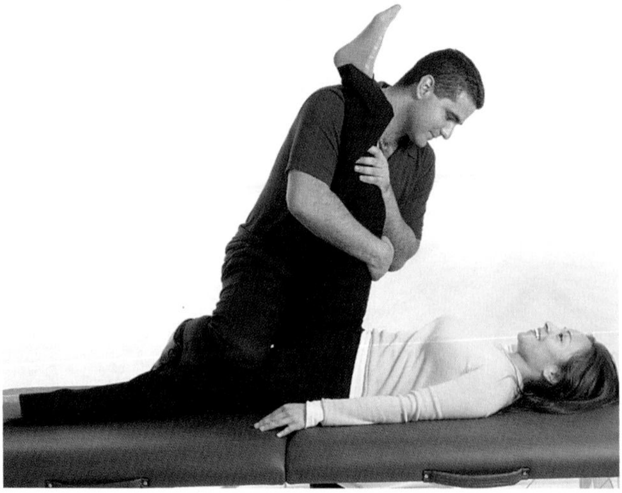

FIGURE 29-3 ■

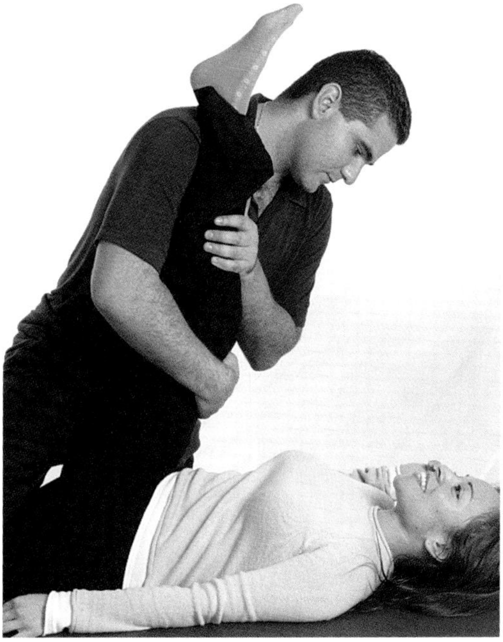

FIGURE 29-4 ■

- Piriformis syndrome
- Sciatica
- Quadriceps dysfunction
- Iliotibial band dysfunction
- Patellofemoral dysfunction

PIRIFORMIS (Figures 29-5 and 29-6)

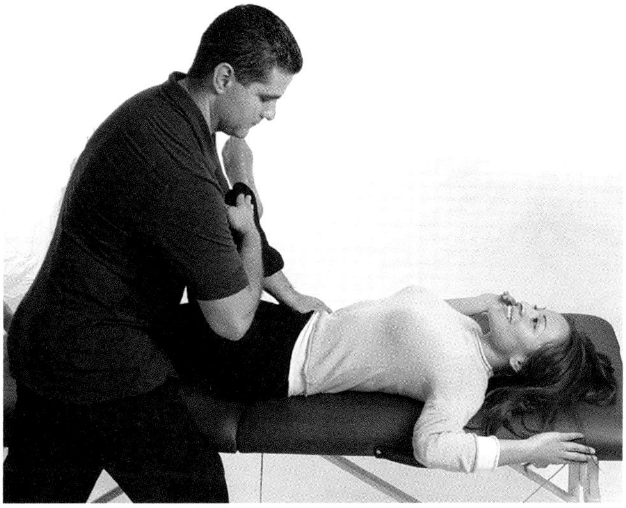

FIGURE 29-5 ■

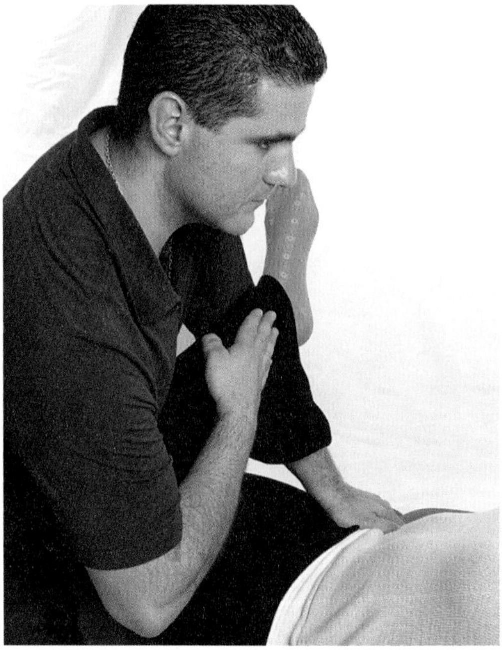

FIGURE 29-6 ■

Can be performed with the following routines:

- Lordosis
- Lower back pain
- Iliopsoas disorder
- Piriformis dysfunction
- Sciatica

ROTATOR CUFF (Figures 29-7 and 29-8)

Can be performed with the following routines:

- Thoracic outlet syndrome
- Frozen shoulder
- Rotator cuff tear

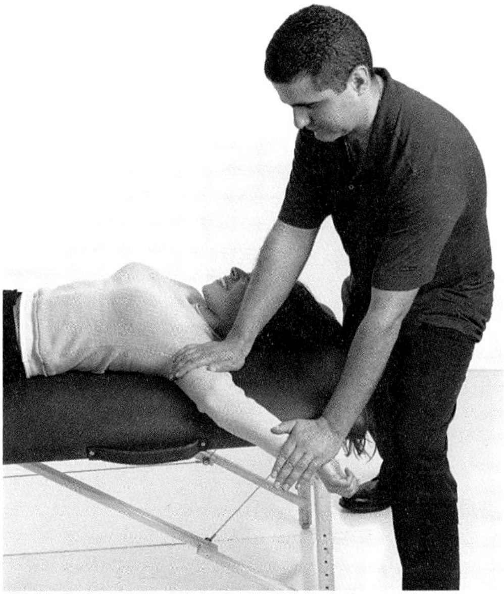

FIGURE 29-7

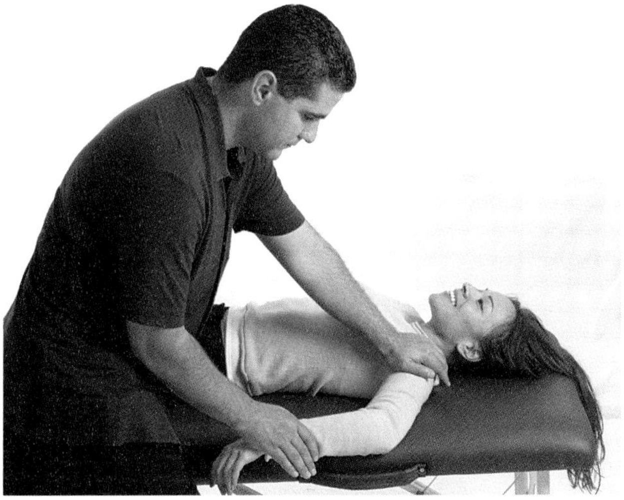

FIGURE 29-8

ILIOPSOAS (Figures 29-9 and 29-10)

Can be performed with the following routines:

- Lower back pain
- Lordosis
- Iliopsoas dysfunction
- Scoliosis
- Quadriceps dysfunction

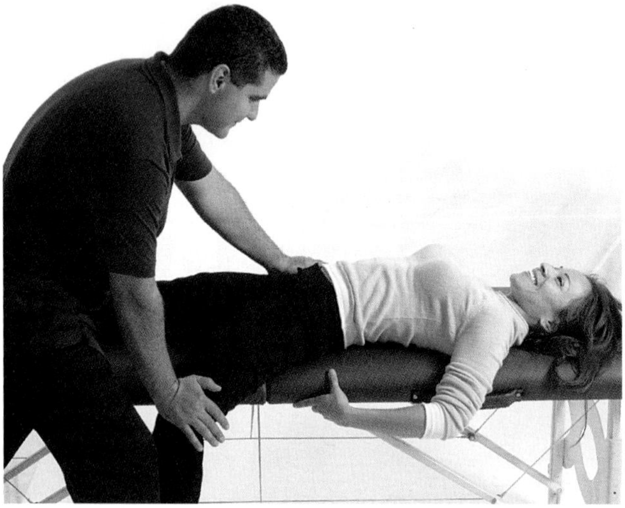

FIGURE 29-9 ■

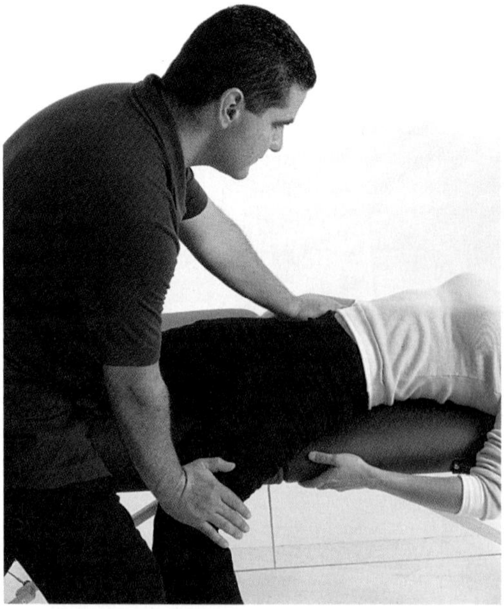

FIGURE 29-10 ■

QUADRICEPS (Figures 29-11 and 29-12)

Can be performed with the following routines:

- Quadriceps dysfunction
- Lower back pain
- Scoliosis
- Lordosis
- Piriformis dysfunction
- Sciatica
- Iliotibial band dysfunction
- Patellofemoral dysfunction

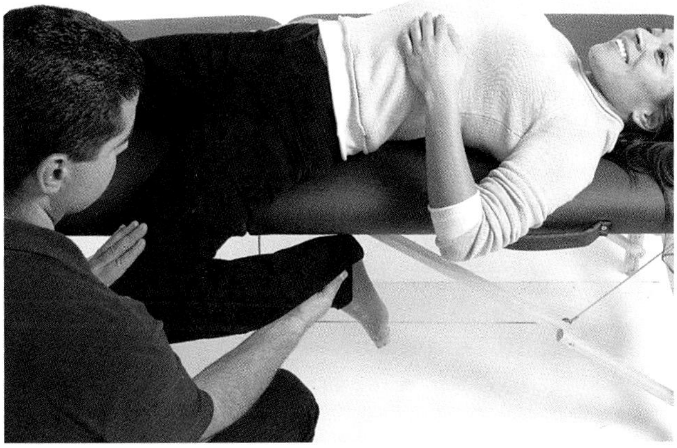

FIGURE 29-11

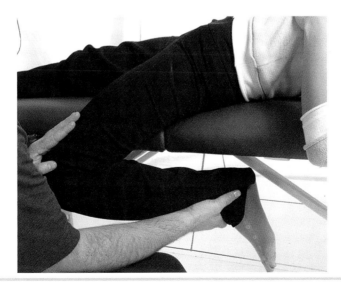

FIGURE 29-12

CERVICAL (Figures 29-13 and 29-14)

Can be performed with the following routines:

- Headaches
- Migraines
- Thoracic outlet syndrome
- Torticollis
- Whiplash
- Rotator cuff tear
- Kyphosis
- Scoliosis

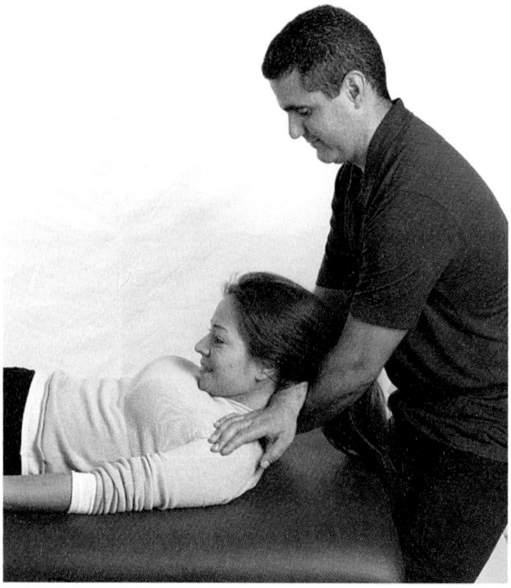

FIGURE 29-13

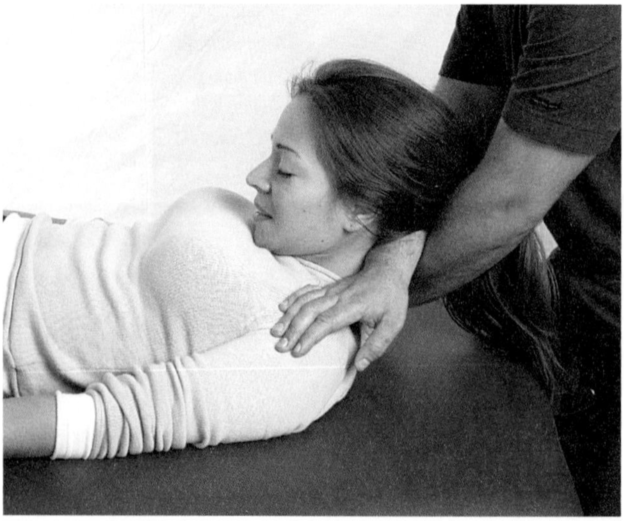

FIGURE 29-14

LATERAL CERVICAL (Figure 29-15)

Can be performed with the following routines:

- Headaches
- Migraines
- Thoracic outlet syndrome
- Torticollis
- Whiplash
- Rotator cuff tear
- Kyphosis
- Scoliosis

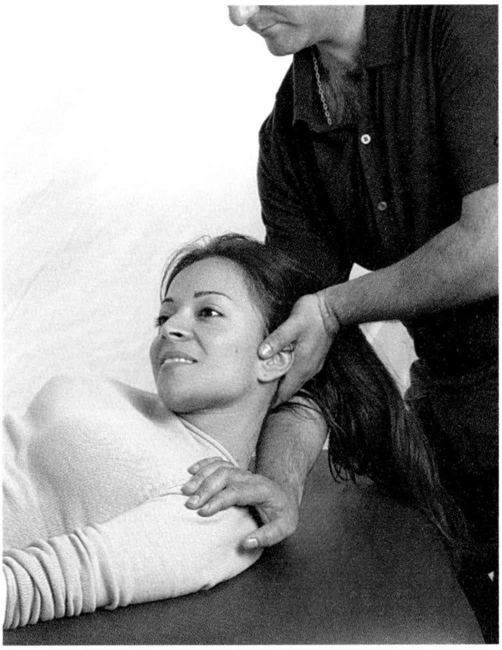

FIGURE 29-15

GASTROCNEMIUS (Figure 29-16)

Can be performed with the following routines:

- Piriformis
- Sciatica
- Quadriceps
- Iliotibial band dysfunction
- Patellofemoral dysfunction
- Shin splints
- Plantar fasciitis

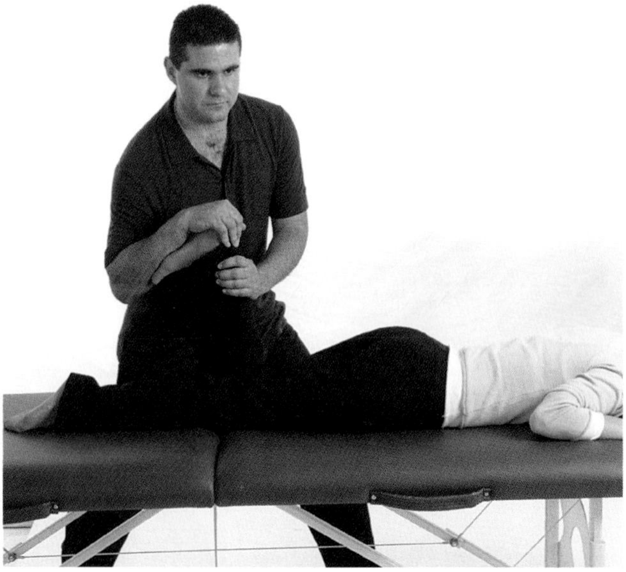

FIGURE 29-16

BACK (Figure 29-17)

Can be performed with the following routines:

- Kyphosis
- Scoliosis
- Lordosis
- Lower back pain

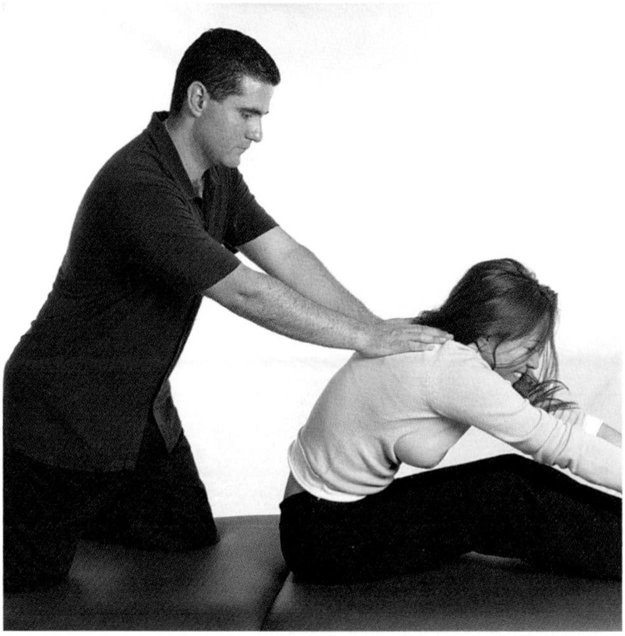

FIGURE 29-17

EXTENSORS OF THE HAND (Figures 29-18 and 29-19)

Can be performed with the following routines:

- Lateral epicondylitis
- Carpal tunnel syndrome

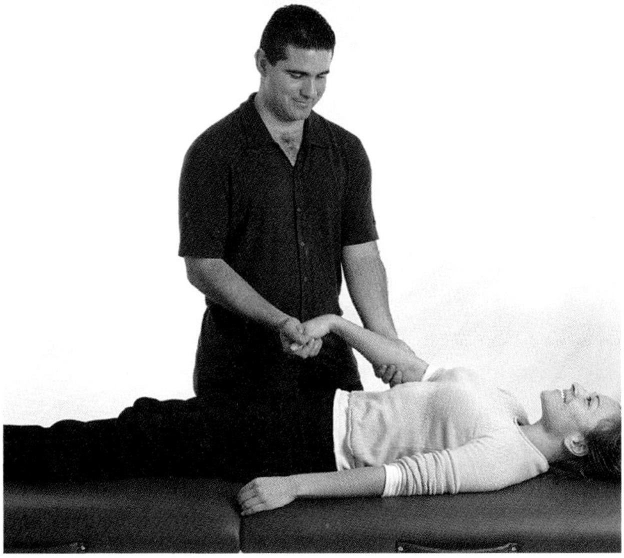

FIGURE 29-18

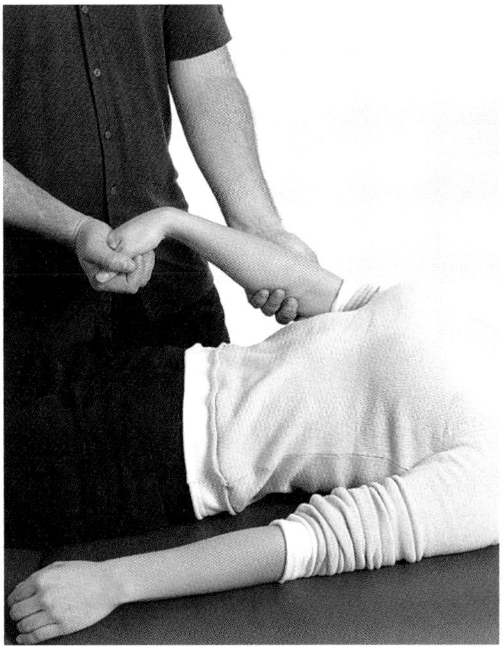

FIGURE 29-19

FLEXORS OF THE HAND (Figure 29-20)

Can be performed with the following routines:

- Medial epicondylitis
- Carpal tunnel syndrome

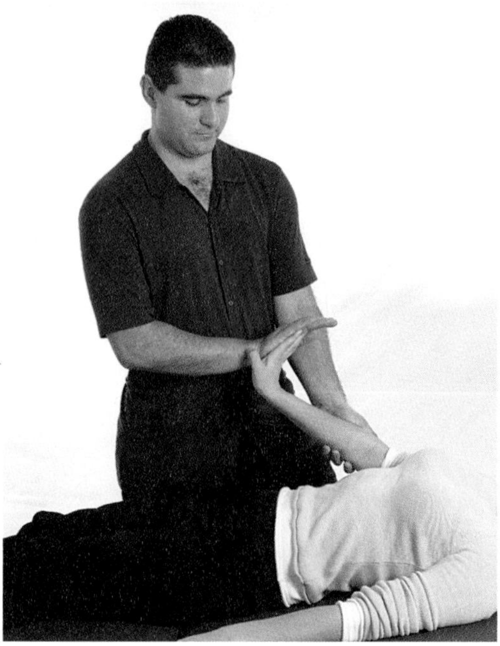

FIGURE 29-20

LOWER BACK (Figures 29-21 and 29-22)

Can be performed with the following routines:

- Lower back pain
- Scoliosis
- Lordosis
- Piriformis dysfunction
- Sciatica
- Iliopsoas dysfunction

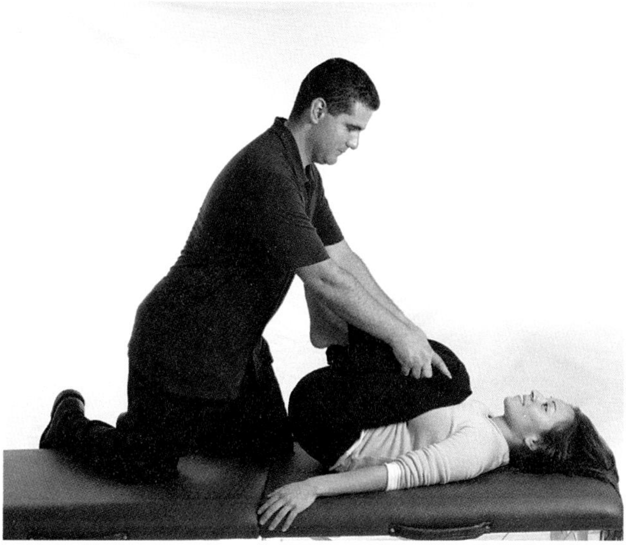

FIGURE 29-21

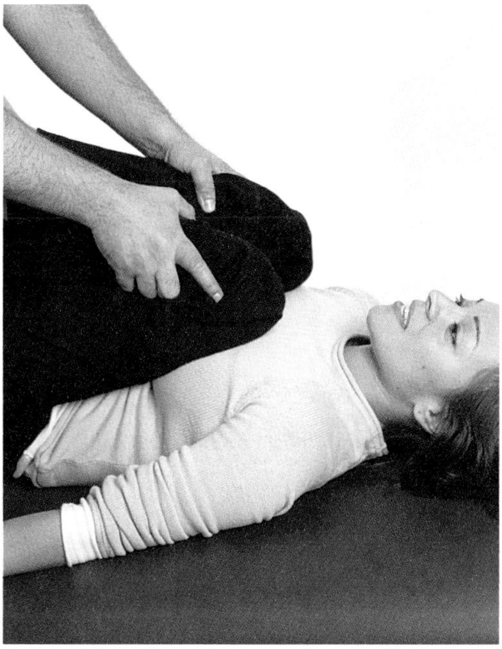

FIGURE 29-22

SACRAL AND LOWER BACK (Figures 29-23, 29-24, 29-25)

Can be performed with the following routines:

- Lower back pain
- Scoliosis
- Lordosis
- Piriformis dysfunction
- Sciatica
- Iliopsoas dysfunction

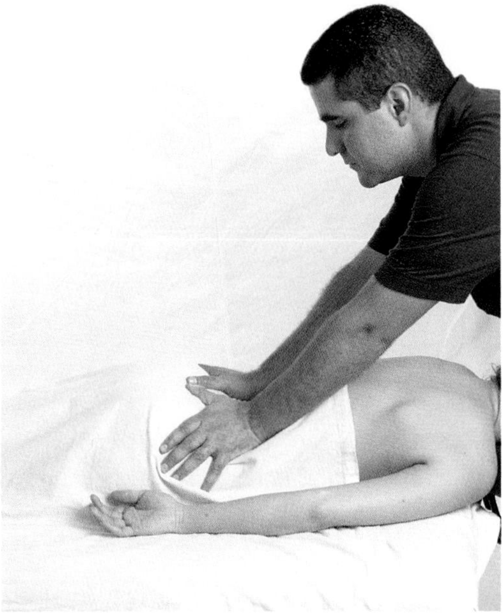

FIGURE 29-23

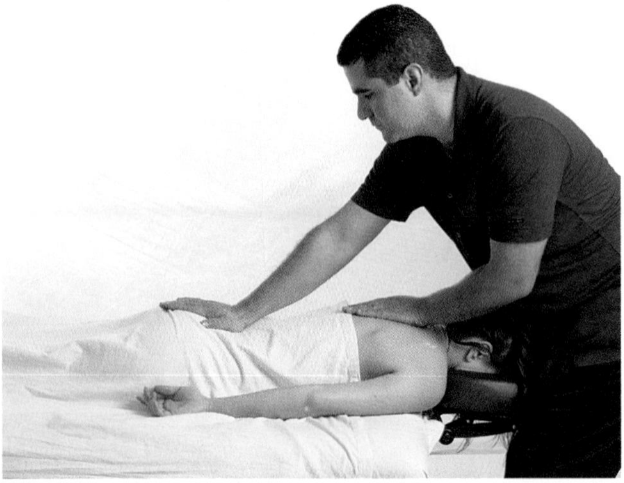

FIGURE 29-24

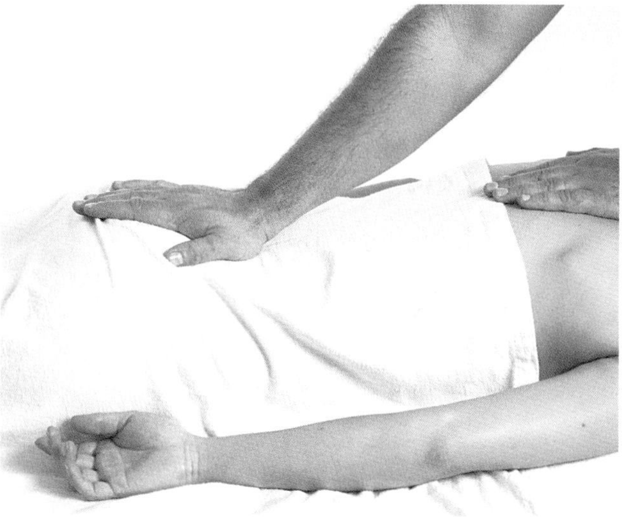

FIGURE 29-25

SIDE-LYING SPINAL STRETCH (Figure 29-26)

Can be performed with the following routines:

- Lower back pain
- Scoliosis
- Lordosis
- Piriformis dysfunction
- Sciatica
- Iliopsoas dysfunction

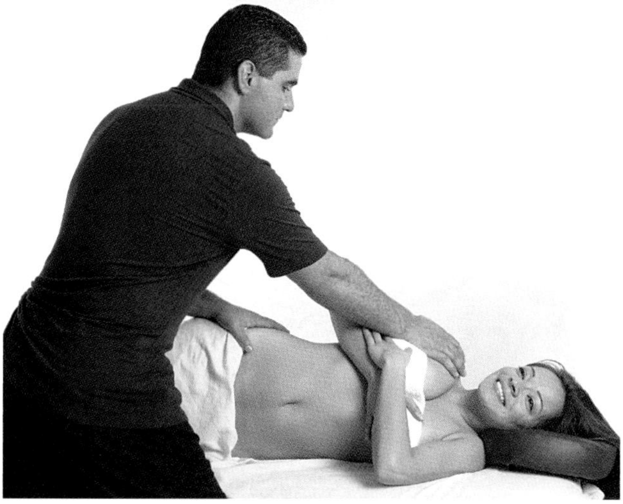

FIGURE 29-26

GLOSSARY

Achondroplasia: An inherited bone growth disorder that may cause dwarfism.

Active trigger point: An area of high nerve facilitation within a taut band of skeletal muscle or associated fascia. The point can either be active or latent. If active it can refer pain to another area.

Ballistic: A type of stretching that includes bouncing. This type of stretching causes micro-tears in the muscle fiber that later develop into scar tissue, reducing ROM in the joint.

Carpal tunnel syndrome: A disorder in which the median nerve is compressed at the wrist causing symptoms such as burning, tingling, numbness in the fingers—especially the thumb, index, and middle fingers—and difficulty gripping or making a fist, which often causes dropping of things.

Cauda equina syndrome: A disorder affecting the bundle of nerve roots (cauda equina) of the lower lumbar region of the spinal cord. This condition can cause sudden bowel and/or bladder incontinence.

Circular friction: Circular friction is often used in an effort to increase hyperemia in an area and is often applied around bony landmarks, such as joints or large bony areas. It can also be used in the treatment of ligaments to increase synovial fluid secretion and aid in breaking up local area adhesions. This technique should be applied using a circular, controlled digital movement. Care should be taken to avoid friction directly on a bone.

Congenital kyphosis: A type of kyphosis. Sometimes the spinal column does not develop properly while the fetus is in utero, resulting in the malformation of bones or the fusing together of several vertebrae. These abnormal situations may lead to progressive kyphosis as the infant grows, and surgical treatment may be needed at a very young age.

Constipation: An obstruction in the large intestine that prohibits the passage of stool through its normal path to the colon for elimination.

Coxalgic gait: In osteoarthritis of the hip, the smooth head of the femur becomes uneven, restricting the motion of the hip joint (the motion of the femoral head in the acetabulum), making the joint restricted and painful. This is especially evident in the swing phase, when the hip and knee have to be flexed to bring the leg forward and in front of the other foot. The hyperextension of the hip at the end of the stance phase may be diminished; hence, the step becomes shorter. To enable the swing-phase leg to clear the ground in a very severe restriction of hip flexion, a person will lift the stance-phase leg up on the toes. The width of the step is reduced, depending on the degree of abduction limitation. Components of the normal gait that may be increased in the painful-knee or coxalgic gait are flexion and extension of the lumbar spine and backward and forward tilting of the pelvis. The lateral shift of the trunk is oftentimes increased, mainly with one-sided hip pain and restriction.

Cross-fiber friction: Cross-fiber friction is generally applied to the muscle belly perpendicular to the muscle fiber, origins, and insertions. As with any other friction technique, cross-fiber friction is correctly applied only when a therapist has a thorough knowledge of the muscular and skeletal system, including muscle origins, insertions, muscle fiber direction, endangerment sites, and bony landmarks.

Cryotherapy: A type of massage using ice in efforts to produce numbing and vasoconstriction.

Deep transverse friction: Popularized by James Cyriax, this method broadens the fibrous tissues of muscles, tendons, or ligaments, breaking down the unwanted fibrous adhesions and thereby restoring mobility to muscles. Although cross-fiber and deep transverse friction are popularly believed to be the same, it is this author's opinion that deep transverse friction can be applied at a deeper level than cross-fiber to a muscle grain, incorporating muscle movement at times, e.g., rotating the forearm at the time of technique application on the extensors of the hand. Deep transverse friction can be applied for as long as 15 minutes to create a controlled re-injury of the tissue, which results in:

1. Restructuring of the connective tissue
2. Increased circulation
3. Temporary analgesia
4. Increased ROM

Diagnosis: A labeling of signs and symptoms by a licensed medical professional.

Discitis: An inflammation of intervertebral disc space.

Ectomorphic: A classification of body type that indicates a thin body.

Endomorphic: A classification of body type that indicates a heavy body.

Erector spinae strain: An injury to either the longissimus spinalis or iliocostalis and can irritate the lower back and increase pain.

Evaluation: A process in which a licensed healthcare practitioner (physician, chiropractor, or therapist) makes a clinical judgment based on information gathered during the interview and examination.

Fascia: A fibrous membrane covering, supporting, and separating muscles; the subcutaneous tissue that connects the skin to the muscles.

Fibromyalgia: A condition characterized by widespread pain in joints, muscles, tendons, and other soft tissues. Symptoms linked with fibromyalgia syndrome (FMS) include fatigue, morning stiffness, sleep problems, headaches, numbness in hands and feet, depression, and anxiety. The most common are disabling fatigue, persistent muscle and joint pain, and severe problems of forgetfulness, irritability, and depression. This condition is more common in women than in men and generally occurs between the ages of 35 and 60; however, there have been cases where FMS has started in the teenage years. Treatments include low-dose drugs, exercise, visualization, massage therapy, counseling, stress management, and support groups.

Flexed-hip gait: In general, individuals who have flexion contractures of the hip-joint capsule have flexed-hip joint. Hip flexion contracture is frequently found in individuals who must sit for long periods of time due to pain in the lower extremities. Hip-joint dysfunction can also be caused by nerve compression, impingement, or neuromuscular dysfunction, among other causes.

Friction: The application of deep movement with the digits, palm, knuckle, or elbow on a soft tissue in an effort to break up adhesions, scar tissue, or nodules that restrict blood flow, range of motion (ROM), movement, or sensation to that area. Friction is intended for soft tissue application and should never be applied directly to a bony landmark.

Most common friction techniques include:

- Cross-fiber friction
- Deep transverse friction
- Circular friction
- Palm friction
- With-fiber friction

Frozen shoulder: A tear or strain in the rotator cuff muscles and/or tendons. Degeneration and general wear-and-tear are usually the two major causes for injury. Because tendons of the rotator cuff muscles receive very little oxygen and nutrients from blood supply, they are especially vulnerable to degeneration with aging; hence, it is common for the elderly to have shoulder problems. This lack of blood supply is also the reason why a shoulder injury can take a long time to heal. There are two common symptoms of a shoulder injury: pain and weakness. Pain is not always felt when a shoulder injury occurs, but most people who feel pain report that it is a very vague pain that can be hard to pinpoint. The earlier a shoulder injury is treated the better. The first 48 to 72 hours, sub-acute stage, are crucial to a complete and speedy recovery.

Gait cycle: The term *gait cycle* refers to the cyclical pattern of activity that occurs during gait. The gait cycle consists of one stride, which is composed of two steps. Each step of a foot contains a stance phase when the foot is on the ground and a swing phase when the foot is (swinging) in the air.

Headache: Headaches can be caused by trauma, injury, stress, poor sleeping pattern or position, prolonged use of a computer, poor ergonomics, poor posture, a trapped nerve caused by a bulge in one of the discs between the vertebrae, or arthritis of the neck. Pain can range from very mild to severe.

Heel-strike: Heel-strike is a landmark of the gait cycle and is defined as the moment that a person heel strikes—makes contact with—the ground. Heel-strike is the landmark that begins stance phase and ends swing phase.

Hemiplegic gait: Often seen in elderly clients, this gait is usually caused by neurological accidents, such as stroke. Spasticity often appears in four to six weeks after the stroke, resulting in a partial or complete loss of movement and often resulting in severe gait deviations. When the hemiplegia is on the right side, arm swing on the right is lost. The client's arm dangles if it is flaccid, or it stays in a flexed-elbow position if spasticity has set in. To clear the ground during the swing phase, the hip has to be abducted as trunk flexion of the healthy side assists in gaining some elevation and momentum of the pelvis on the affected side. In this case there is minimal stride, and the client walks on the outside of the affected foot, preventing the heel from touching the ground. In an effort to thrust the other leg forward, a person often pushes up on the healthy side by elevating the heel, resulting in further damage and degeneration to the foot, leg, hip, and spine.

Iliopsoas disorder: The iliopsoas is the most important active postural or stabilizing muscle of the hip joint, and a hip flexor. Studies have shown that the iliopsoas made up for paralyzed abductor muscles when it was attached to the greater trochanter, proving that stability to the pelvis was more important than the reduction of hip flexor power. Any weakening or shortening of the iliopsoas will most likely result in lower back pain.

Iliotibial band disorder: An inflammatory condition that is the result of friction (rubbing) of the band of the iliotibial (IT) tendon over the outer bone (femur). Although the syndrome may be caused by direct injury to the knee, it is most often caused by the stress of long-term overuse (e.g., from sports training). Symptoms include an ache or burning sensation at the side of the knee during activity, pain radiating from the lateral hip down to the lateral aspect of the knee. A "snap" may also be felt when the knee is bent and then straightened. Methods of treatment include massage therapy, stretching, rest, or surgery.

Inactive trigger point: An inactive trigger point does not show local tenderness or refer pain when compressed; excess trigger-point stimulation might activate this trigger point.

Intervention: Purposeful and skilled interaction of the therapist with the patient and, when appropriate, other individuals also involved in the patient's care using various methods and techniques to produce changes in the condition that are consistent with the diagnosis and prognosis.

Interview: The thorough questioning of a client to determine any injuries or illness.

Irritated nerve roots: A condition which can irritate the lower back and increase pain.

Ischemic compression: Pressure applied by therapist.

Kyphosis: An exaggerated anterior concave curvature of the thoracic spine. The term *kyphosis* (ki-foe-sis) is usually applied to the curve that results in an exaggerated "round-back." Spinal x-rays allow physicians to measure the degree of the kyphotic curve. Any kyphotic curve that is more than 50 degrees is considered abnormal.

Latent trigger point: A latent trigger point only exhibits pain when compressed and does not refer pain; may or may not radiate pain around the point.

Lateral epicondylitis (tennis elbow): An inflammation or degeneration of the tendon that attaches to the lateral epicondyle of the humerus; an injury that is common among tennis players as a result of poor backhand technique or a too-small grip. A too-small grip means the muscles in the elbow must work harder, and they eventually become inflamed. The majority of people who get tennis elbow are between 40 and 50 years old, but it can affect athletes or non-athletes of any age. The symptoms for this injury are very similar to the entrapment of the radial nerve. Common treatments include the use of ultrasound or laser, massage therapy, rehabilitation, anti-inflammatory medication, steroid injection, or surgery (for pain lasting more than one year).

Lordosis: An abnormal anterior convex curvature of the lumbar spine (swayback). Lordosis (lor-doe-sis) can also be found in the neck (cervical), but it is most common in the lumbar region. A lumbar lordosis can be painful, sometimes affecting movement, posture, spinal integrity, and internal organs.

Lumbago: Pain in the lower back.

Medial epicondylitis (golfer's elbow): An inflammation or degeneration of the tendon that attaches to the medial epicondyle of the humerus. This injury can be caused by a forceful and repeated bending of the wrist and fingers, causing tiny ruptures of the muscle and tendon in this area. Common causes for this injury include golfing, repeated bending of the wrist, gripping, grasping, and turning the hand (overuse). Symptoms include tenderness and pain at the medial epicondyle, which is worsened by flexing the wrist. Common treatments include the use of anti-inflammatory medications, massage therapy, injections, and surgery. Often, resting the area prevents further injury while allowing time to heal. Medial epicondylitis can be avoided by taking frequent breaks during work or play to improve overall arm muscle condition, and limiting heavy pushing, pulling, or grasping.

Mesomorphic: A classification of body type which indicates a muscular body.

Mid-stance: Midstance is the midpoint of the stance phase of the gait cycle.

Migraine: A headache that is usually very intense and disabling. Migraine headaches can be neurological, neuromuscular, vascular, or nutritional in nature. The word *migraine* originates from the Greek word *hemikranion* (pain affecting one side of the head).

Myofascial dysfunction: An abnormal fascia condition that causes the development of poor posture or structural misalignment and could result in the displacement of bones or the entrapment of blood vessels and nerves. Myofascial release (MFR) is known as a deep tissue technique that addresses the fascia and surrounding tissue that connects all muscles, bones, and internal organs.

Nonstructural scoliosis: A type of scoliosis that involves a curve in the spine, without rotation, that could be reversible.

Obesity: Excess weight, which may cause some overweight people to lean backward to improve balance, thereby creating an exaggerated lordotic curvature.

Osteoporosis: A bone density disease that may cause vertebrae to lose strength, compromising the spine's structural integrity.

Outcomes: Result of patient pain management, which includes remediation of functional limitation and disability and optimization of patient satisfaction, including primary or secondary prevention.

Painful-knee gait: To protect an injured knee, a person will unconsciously contract the quadriceps to suppress any motion in the knee. The client therefore assumes an outward rotation of the affected extremity, resulting in a duck-like walk. The medial aspect of the leg and foot are pointed in the direction of forward motion. Therefore flexion and extension in the knee are avoided, and the entire sole of the foot can be placed on the ground, potentially resulting in an increased rotation of the pelvis.

Palm friction: Palm friction can be applied with one or two hands and is not intended to be applied as deeply as deep transverse friction. This technique is typically used on large muscle areas (e.g., quadriceps, latissimus dorsi, or trapezius) to increase circulation to a large area, break up superficial adhesions, increase blood flow, and increase tissue pliability.

Parkinson's gait: Parkinson's disease has a major effect on the central nervous system and on a person's gait. Most often found in elderly individuals, this ailment is often treated with drug therapy. A person who has Parkinson's disease stands with a slightly forward-flexed trunk and flexed knees and hips; there is often a continuous tremor throughout the body. In ambulation (walking), there is usually no arm swing and the trunk swings from right to left in a block motion. Gait deviation depends upon severity, intensity, and persistence of the disease.

Patellofemoral dysfunction: Results from an injury that occurs at the articulation between the patella (kneecap) and the underlying femur. The patella is a diamond-shaped bone that lies in an identically shaped groove in front of the femur. The patella functions as a pulley to assist the quadriceps by providing a mechanical advantage for added strength. Patellofemoral dysfunction may occur when the patella is forced with excessive pressure against the underlying femur or when it rubs excessively on one side of the groove. This causes an irritation of the cartilage of the patella, resulting in inflammation and pain.

Patient history: A thorough patient history must be taken to determine the type of massage treatment best suited for the individual. Questions about the type of work they do, accidents they have suffered, first pain occurrence, and physical sensations are all pieces of a larger puzzle waiting to be completed.

Piriformis syndrome (sciatica): A condition in which the piriformis muscle irritates the sciatic nerve, causing pain in the buttocks and referring pain along the course of the sciatic nerve (back of the thigh). Patients generally complain of pain deep in the buttocks, which is aggravated by sitting, climbing stairs, or performing squats.

Plantar fasciitis: An inflammation of the plantar fascia, a thin layer of tough tissue supporting the arch of the foot. Repeated microscopic tears of the plantar fascia cause discomfort, pain, and scar tissue. This disorder is also referred to as "heel spurs"; however, this is not always accurate because bony growths on the heel may or may not be a factor.

Postural kyphosis: A type of kyphosis, often attributed to "slouching." It is an exaggerated increase of the natural curve of the thoracic spine, which usually becomes noticeable during adolescence. More common among girls than boys.

Prognosis: Determination of the level of optimal improvement that might be attained through intervention and the amount of time required to reach that level.

Proprioceptive neuromuscular facilitation (PNF) technique: Proprioceptive neuromuscular facilitation (PNF) stretching is a type of muscle stretching that utilizes the proprioceptive neurologic golgi tendon organ reflex to facilitate the stretch (hence the name). A PNF stretch is performed by having the client actively isometrically contract (against your resistance) the muscle that you want to stretch. After the isometric contraction, ask the client to relax the muscle and you can then stretch the muscle further than you would have been able to otherwise. PNF stretching is also known as CR (contract-relax) stretching or PIR (post-isometric relaxation) stretching. (Note: the term *PNF stretching* is actually applicable to a broader category of stretching than the specific CR stretch that was just described; however, the term *PNF* is widely used by people to specifically refer to this type of stretch.)

Push-off: The final movement in the stance phase of the gait cycle, when the heel of the leg lifts from the ground and the ball of the foot pushes the body forward. At this moment, the body is propelled forward by the action of the calf muscles and hyperextension of the hip.

Quadriceps dysfunction: A condition known to cause weakness, paresthesia, reduced knee and hip range of motion (ROM), and cramping. This dysfunction could be the result of trauma, inactivity, overuse, strains, or other thigh-related ailments. Symptoms include numbness, a tingling feeling, knee pain, and cramping. There are four muscles that compose the quadriceps group, but only one (rectus femoris) crosses the hip joint and is vulnerable to injury.

Range of motion: Movement of joints.

Rotator cuff tear: A tear in one of the four rotator cuff muscles or their tendons. The four muscles, supraspinatus, infraspinatus, teres minor, and subscapularis (SITS) originate from the scapula and together form a single tendon unit that form a "cuff" over the upper end of the arm (head of the humerus). The rotator cuff helps to lift and rotate the arm and to stabilize the ball of the humerus within the joint. Symptoms of a rotator cuff tear may develop acutely or have a more gradual onset. Acute trauma is usually brought on by a lifting injury or a fall on the affected arm; however, onset is gradual and may be caused by repetitive activity or by degeneration of the tendon. A client with a rotator cuff tear might feel pain in the front of the shoulder that radiates down the side of the arm. Other symptoms may include stiffness, loss of motion, and loss of range of motion (ROM).

Sacroiliac gait: Motion between the sacrum and the iliac bone can be observed during normal gait. Both bones are firmly connected to each other. However, some motion during walking occurs in this area. Individuals who have any affliction or disorder in the sacroiliac joint tend to walk slightly bent forward with decreased motion of the pelvis. This results in restricted pelvic movement, followed by shorter steps.

Scheuermann's kyphosis: A type of kyphosis. Named after the Danish radiologist who first described the condition, it presents significantly worse cosmetic deformity than postural kyphosis. Scheuermann's (shoe-er-mans) kyphosis usually affects the upper (thoracic) spine, but it can also occur in the lower (lumbar) spine. Aggravating factors include heavy physical activity and long periods of standing or sitting.

Scoliosis: A complicated deformity that is characterized by both lateral (side-to-side) curvature and vertebral rotation (torque) of the spine. If the disease is progressive, the vertebrae and spinous processes in the area of the major curve rotate toward the concavity of the deviation. On the concave side of the curve, the ribs rest closely together. On the convex side, they are more separated.

Shin splints (medial tibial stress syndrome): An inflammation of the thin layer of tissue that covers the bone (periosteum). An injury or strain that occurs along or just behind the inner (medial) edge of the shin (tibia). The pain usually spans about 3 to 4 inches. Shin splints result from exercise and overuse of the involved leg(s).

Spinal nerve irritation: A condition that can irritate the lower back and increase pain.

Spinal torquing: A type of stretching that is contraindicated for the spine.

Spondylolisthesis: Occurs when one vertebra slips forward in relation to an adjacent vertebra, usually in the lumbar spine.

Stance phase: The gait cycle is composed of two phases, the stance phase when the foot is on the ground, and the swing phase when the foot is (swinging) in the air. The stance phase of one foot begins with heel-strike of that foot and ends with toe-off of that foot. The stance phase for each foot accounts for 60% of the gait cycle. Generally, when one foot is in stance phase, the other foot is in swing phase (except for the period of double-limb support in which boot feet are on the ground; this explains why each foot is in stance phase for greater than 50% of the gait cycle). The landmarks of stance phase are heel-strike, foot-flat, midstance, heel-off, and toe-off.

Structural scoliosis: The most common type of scoliosis that can cause the spine to rotate.

Swing phase: The gait cycle is composed of two phases: the stance phase when the foot is on the ground, and the swing phase when the foot is (swinging) in the air. The swing phase of one foot begins with toe-off of that foot and ends with heel-strike of that foot; during this time, the foot is swinging through the air, hence the name. The swing phase for each foot accounts for 40% of the gait cycle. When one foot is in swing phase, the other foot is in stance phase (swing phase accounts for less than 50% of the gait cycle because there is a period of double-limb support in which boot feet are on the ground, i.e., both feet are in stance phase). The swing phase is often subdivided into three phases: early swing, mid swing, and late swing.

Temporal mandibular joint disorder: Temporal mandibular joint disorder results when the muscles of mastication and the jaw joint, or temporal mandibular joint (TMJ), are not working together correctly. It is often masked by headaches, migraines, earaches, tenderness of the jaw muscles, or aching facial pain. Further causes can involve accidents such as injuries to the jaw, head, or neck, or diseases such as arthritis. However, factors relating to the teeth and bite, such as teeth grinding and teeth fit, are believed to be common causes of TMJ disorders. In many cases, if they are treated early, TMJ disorders can be successfully eliminated. Some of the most common symptoms of TMJ disorder include:

- Tenderness of the jaw muscles
- Clicking/popping noises when opening or closing the mouth
- Difficulty in opening mouth
- Lock jaw
- Pain brought on by yawning, chewing, or opening the mouth widely
- Certain types of headaches or neck aches
- Pain in or around the ear often spreading to the face

Thoracic outlet syndrome: A compression, injury, or irritation to the neurovascular structures located at the root of the neck or upper thoracic region (thoracic outlet).

This disorder is often the result of entrapment of the neurovascular structures by the anterior and middle scalene muscles between the clavicle and first rib, possible hypotrophy or hypertrophy of the subclavius, or entrapment by the pectoralis minor muscle.

Torticollis (wryneck): A congenital or acquired condition of limited neck motion in which the person holds the head to one side with the chin pointing to the opposite side. It is the result of the shortening of the sternocleidomastoid (SCM) muscle. In early infancy, a firm, nontender mass may be felt in the belly of the muscle and if left untreated, it can lead to permanent limitation of range of motion (ROM). Symptoms can last for as long as three weeks. Treatments for torticollis are gentle stretching exercises, injections, pain killers, or massage therapy.

Transient structural scoliosis: A type of scoliosis.

Trigger point: An area of high-nerve facilitation that is hyperirritable and painful when compressed, which may result in muscle dysfunction and/or chronic condition.

Whiplash: Soft-tissue injury to the neck that can also be known as neck sprain or neck strain. It is characterized by a set of symptoms that occur after damage to the neck, usually because of sudden extension and flexion (e.g., such as in a rear-end car accident). Injury can involve intervertebral joints, discs, ligaments, cervical muscles, and nerve roots. Neck pain may not be present at the time of the accident but can appear soon after.

With-fiber friction: With-fiber friction, also known as stripping or spreading, is generally applied to the length of the parallel muscle. Aside from increasing circulation, breaking up scar tissue, and realigning muscle fibers, this technique is commonly used to treat nodules (knots). In an effort to treat knots, therapists often mistakenly use techniques such as cross-fiber, circular friction, and direct pressure; however, these techniques only aggravate and increase pain to the area. To understand the reasoning behind the benefit of using with-fiber friction, nodule composition must be understood.

INDEX